Look
Feeli

C000318575

Looking Good, Feeling Great

Rosemary Conley

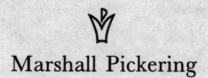

Marshall Pickering

Marshall Pickering
Marshall Morgan and Scott
34–42 Cleveland Street, London, W1P 5FB. U.K.

Cover photograph of Rosemary Conley by Tony Smith

ISBN: 0 551 01835 6

Text Set in Baskerville by Avocet-Robinson, Buckingham.
Printed in Great Britain by Cox & Wyman, Reading

Contents

Acknowledgments

My grateful thanks to Tim Lacey of Keith Hall Salons for his valuable help and expertise in the compilation of the haircare section of this book.

My thanks also to IPC Magazines Ltd. for their permission to reprint material from my earlier books.

I would also like to say a special 'thank you' to my secretary Diane Stevens for her hard work and co-operation in the preparation of my manuscript and of course to my husband, Mike, for his devoted support and help at all times.

Introduction

Since writing my *Hip and Thigh Diet*, followed by the *Complete Hip and Thigh Diet*, I feel I have made literally hundreds of new friends. These are the many, many women who have written to me to say that my diet has worked for them and that, for many, after years of trying (in some cases),they at last felt like new people. For instance, Doris Langley wrote to me saying how she felt – 'I feel I know you more as a personal friend now rather than just someone who really helped me through a very depressing period through being overweight. It opened up a whole new life for me, full of confidence and healthier in every aspect, and more than anything, I'm so pleased with my new eating habits.' There was Lorna Cowley who, after losing a lot of weight on the *Hip and Thigh Diet*, took up driving after 25 years. There are so many stories like this. I must say it was wonderful to hear such encouraging stories from my readers. So many were just looking for that little bit of courage to start after suffering disappointment after disappointment with diets that only succeeded in reducing their bank balances! I received literally hundreds of letters and I replied personally to every single one. It is for all these women who found new hope and confidence through my *Hip and Thigh Diet* books that this book is written. *Looking Good and Feeling Great* is about the way we *look* and the way we *are*. Health and beauty aren't ends in themselves; our ultimate goal is *happiness* and this needs to radiate from within. No amount of dieting, exercising, new clothes or make-up styles will alter us if we're basically unhappy. This book, I hope, will help you maximise not just your looks, but your life! But first let me tell you how it works for me.

For 17 years I have enjoyed helping women look and feel better about themselves. It began in a very small way when I formed my first slimming club in my kitchen in the early 1970 s. I invited half-a-dozen of my neighbours to join me once a week when I issued a diet, weighed them and gave talks on making the most of themselves. I had just finished a course of good grooming and modelling and was fascinated at the difference it made to how I felt about *myself*. All of a sudden I felt I was wearing my clothes properly and applying my make-up so that it minimised my bad points and enhanced my better ones. I felt so much happier as a person as a result. I felt I wanted to share this with others and hopefully improve the quality of their lives too. From that very small beginning and the successful loss of weight and improvement in appearance of my tiny class, we ventured into our local Village Hall where we opened a class to the general public three months later. Twenty-nine eager ladies joined on that first night and, for the first time in my life, I felt I was doing something really useful. Six months later, I gave up my job as a secretary and opened three more clubs around Leicestershire. Within eight years I had fifty classes held throughout my county of Leicestershire, with many lecturers taking classes on my behalf.

Then I was invited to meet a rather formidable but very charming lady, Jane Reed, who suggested that a magazine she published – *Successful Slimming* – would like to expand into the slimming club market and would I like to run the operation? I was totally overwhelmed by the suggestion and gave it considerable thought. I felt it was the opportunity of a lifetime and considered I should certainly 'have a go'. In three years the network of clubs had grown to 600, with 400 lecturers doing their best to help overweight ladies in the UK to slim their bodies and to make the most of their appearance. Life in the fast lane was fun for a while – I even enjoyed the wheeling and dealing, internal politics, and working all hours. Unfortunately, however, all work and no play took its toll on my marriage and it was mutually decided by my husband, Phil, and me, that we should go our separate ways. I bought a pleasant house on the outskirts of Leicester and my daughter stayed with me at weekends and with Phil during the week.

Moving out on my own made me more aware of my Creator and I certainly became more dependent on him. I was brought up in a church-going family, but I had never really understood what Christianity was all about. In fact it hadn't meant very much to me, but now I began to discover that God was really the only real, 100 per cent trustworthy friend I had. I began to 'talk' to him. I would discuss situations, ask his advice and felt strangely supported in my decision to go it alone.

Although we both enjoyed great friendship and respect for each other, our marriage basically wasn't right. I can remember crying down the phone to Phil on the evening that I had left and saying 'I don't know why I've left, but I just know I had to – something, somebody, has told me I must.'

As the months went on our torn emotions began to heal and we settled into our new, independent lifestyles.

We both buried ourselves in our work and began to make new friends. I worked very long hours and the business was growing by the day. I decided to take a much-needed weekend break and went pony-trekking in South Wales with some friends. Mike was a new member of the group and he seemed a friendly, genuine sort of a guy and was very good-looking. My heart sank, however, when I discovered he was only 23 – I was 36. I had been out with younger men before, but had never taken those relationships too seriously. Mike was different. We arranged to meet again a week or so after the trekking escapade and would have spent an enjoyable and relaxing evening together except that my new German Shepherd pup had tummy troubles and kept unloading her problems on to my brand new plain beige carpet right in front of us! Mike, who is exceptionally good with animals, amazingly endeared himself to my four-legged companion, while I cleared the mess away. Nick, the pup, in fact was to play a very important part in cementing our relationship.

Every month we held a Board meeting in London and as Managing Director of the clubs, I always had to attend. It involved staying overnight in a hotel and of course this created problems with the pup. Having asked everyone I could think of to have Nick for a night I drew a complete blank. In desperation, I rang Mike who willingly agreed to dog-sit while I was away. Mike and I got on famously from then on and before long Mike moved in with me. He was totally understanding of my work pressures and when we did have time together we enjoyed a lot of fun and laughter.

I had always felt that if I found anyone I wanted to live with I should sell my house and move to a new place which we could develop as our own home.

Together we looked at many houses, but they really weren't at all what we were seeking. Then we saw and advertisement for an old parsonage in a village just north of Leicester. It was very large and grand and appeared to be in quite good order. It was cheap because it was a bit of a 'white elephant'. Situated anywhere else it would have been a perfect family home, but with a trunk road running just outside the front door and a river and weir at the bottom of the garden, the house was plagued with hazards for a family. We wouldn't be able to have children because I had had a hysterectomy and my daughter Dawn was now old enough and sensible enough to cope with the traffic anyway. We fell in love with the house immediately. A surveyor friend gave it the once-over and told us about the many things that needed doing. We were undeterred and

10

bought it. It was an ambitious project, but we felt we were meant to have it. We sold the other house in a week and we had moved into a little caravan in the new back garden while the damp-proofing, rewiring and woodworm treatment were completed. It was early December and we huddled in that caravan with icicles on the inside of the windows! We both went to work each day and worked on the house in the evenings and at weekends and moved in for Christmas. In just a year the majority of the work was done to transform it into a home. Help came from all kinds of quarters. For example, the workmen did more than we had asked of them, but charged the same price. We found we were eligible for grants for all kinds of things – it was staggering how we got it all done. Through all these events, I felt that God was drawing me closer and closer to himself.

However, the business was going through a bad patch and the classes were not making enough to pay the ever increasing level of expenses. The parent company was having difficulties too, coping with a strike which cost them millions. My board of directors were gloomy and as Managing Director, quite rightly, I carried the can for the clubs. It was a horrible period of my life and Mike was marvellous. The possibility of the clubs' closure was discussed, but I felt certain in my own mind that we could turn the business round. We changed our methods of trading on to a franchise basis, but this was fraught with problems. My lecturers were not entrepreneurs – they were women who just wanted to earn a bit of extra money without any risk to themselves. They couldn't see that on the franchise scheme they could earn a great deal more than they had in the past. Despite many initial problems little by little we managed to rebuild the business and reached a satisfactory trading position. Nevertheless, all the hassle had left its mark on me and I decided that I definitely wouldn't renew my contract.

At this point, amazingly, the way ahead again became plain, though not in the way I would have chosen. The magazine with whom we had been associated was sold. The new owners insisted that the name of our clubs should be changed so as not to appear connectd with their new acquisition. It would not have been too difficult to change the name though it would have involved a lot of expense in re-printing all our stationery, but our lease on our Head Office was due to expire in twelve months and I had made known to my other directors that I had no wish to continue with the company long-term. So it was decided that the only practical solution was to disband the company that Spring and words cannot express adequately the relief that I felt when I realised I could now be my own boss again. However, it was Christmas and I was the only one in my organisation to know what was planned; whilst I was relieved it was all going to be over I did feel for my staff who had worked so well for me for many years. Redundancy is a terrible blow for anyone, but my staff were very special and I dreaded telling them. So, I decided to let them have a good Christmas, unaware of the plans for the following Spring. For me, leaving an executive job, a good steady salary and a company car, proved a daunting prospect and our biggest liability had to go. So, our beautiful home was put on the market. The property was now in perfect condition and looked good. Lots of potential buyers enthused at the spaciousness and the many elegant features of what had once been Mountsorrel Hall before it had been bought by the Church about a hundred years ago. However, restrictive covenants hindered potential commercial buyers and we were getting nowhere.

With all these problems simmering in the background, Mike and I had been experiencing a few problems in our relationship and we decided that we should go our separate ways. Mike bought a cottage in the next village and moved out just after Christmas. I had until the end of March to wind up the company and I looked forward to a simple life in a country cottage, with the dogs (by now Nick had had pups and we had kept the quiet one, Sheba) and George the cat.

Mike and I stayed the best of friends and we still saw each other weekly. I was invited to his cottage for dinner on his birthday. I remember we spent most of the evening in tears! We still loved each other and yet I wanted to be free. Looking back I'm not surprised I was a bit mixed up.

Then I became very ill. What seemed like a serious kidney infection turned out to be a gall bladder problem and I was confined to bed for five days. My body temperature varied from what seemed like boiling point to ten degrees below freezing! I felt *so* ill. Mike came back to nurse me and was wonderful. The doctor called daily and the massive dose of antibiotics he prescribed plus a very low fat diet seemed to sort me out. It was now six weeks before the closedown of the business. I went back to work on the Monday and caught a bad cold immediately. My mouth was covered in sores and I lost my voice. Back to the doctor I went to be told to eat lots of sweets in an attempt to regain my voice. Without thinking, I ate some butterscotch forgetting that the butter content would in turn aggravate the gall stone problem again. The next day the awful pain that I had experienced the week before, returned. I strictly kept off all fat for the next few days, but on the Saturday morning I got out of bed, went to the bathroom feeling dreadful and collapsed when I returned to the bedroom. Mike called the ambulance thinking I had died as I had turned green! I was rushed into hospital where various doctors puzzled over my condition. After causing the inevitable havoc by collapsing several times in casualty, I was put on a saline drip and soon felt much better. While I underwent numerous tests to establish the real problem, I can remember lying in bed and saying 'I know you have a plan for our lives God, but I think your timing for me to be ill now is positively lousy! What good can possibly come from this?'

Leading the busy life that I did I rarely had time to read books or magazines, but stuck in a hospital bed I *did* have time for a luxurious pastime so I bought a woman's magazine. A photograph of Cliff Richard attracted me to an advertisement for a book called *Power for Living*. It was free to anyone who completed and returned the coupon and it explained how, with God's help, anyone could enjoy the kind of power for living experienced by Cliff and other eminent and highly successful people pictured in the advertisement.

As I lay in my hospital bed, helpless, ill and with five weeks before closedown, if anyone needed power for living I felt I did! I posted the coupon.

Eventually, the specialist suggested I should go home and return in three weeks to have my gall bladder removed. 'It's quite a simple operation' he remarked casually, 'and you'll be out of action for about six weeks.' I took my courage in both hands and said 'Well, that's very kind of you, but I really can't do that just at the moment.' I explained the situation with the business and my exercise classes which would, after the company folded, be my only means of income. If I stopped taking them for six weeks, they too would be non-existent. Not surprisingly, he didn't sympathise with my dilemma, telling me that if I wanted to live my life on a tightrope wondering when next I was going to collapse, that was up to me, but I was being very silly! I promised that I would follow a virtually fat-free diet thus avoiding the problem for at least the next few weeks, then we would see how things progressed. He did, however, insist on further tests to establish exactly how bad my gall stones were.

It was on the morning of one of these visits to out-patients that my *Power for Living* book arrived. As I sat in the hospital having swallowed some foul tasting liquid that was to illuminate my gall bladder, I fed on every word I read in my new book. It was fascinating. It told how some very famous people had experienced terrible circumstances, but had found tremendous strength and help in God. It went on to explain in simple understandable terms what

14

Christianity was about: that Jesus is the bridge between us and God, and that to those who invite him into the centre of their lives, God, by his Holy Spirit 'takes up residence' as it were helping and guiding at all times, enabling us to live life to the full and giving meaning and purpose to all we do. It all seemed to fall into place for me. I couldn't wait to get home to read more.

Mike by now had returned to his cottage so I was all alone when I returned from the hospital. I had my evening meal and went to bed early so I could read more of my new book. I was riveted. It seemed to be written just for me.

At the end of the book there was a prayer which summed up my situation perfectly. It went along the lines of 'Lord I have not been very good at organising or running my life. I would like to give my life to you. Please come into my life, my body and my soul and take over.'

I got out of bed and prayed this prayer for all I was worth. I meant every single word from the bottom of my heart. Trying to go to sleep after that was useless. I couldn't. I felt positively glowing in my heart, in my head and to the tips of my toes! My mind danced with a new sense of purpose and direction. I tossed and turned but sleep was the furthest thing from my mind. At 1.30 a.m. I switched on the light. Out came a notebook and I began to list my plans. After a few calculations I decided there was a good chance that I could afford to keep my home after all, if the Lord thought I should. I dearly longed for my own horse – the realisation of a life-long ambition – and I decided one could be accommodated within the grounds of the house. Everything was suddenly *so* exciting.

The next day a new boyfriend was coming to dinner. As soon as he arrived I bombarded him with all that had happened to me the night before. The poor chap must have wondered what had hit him! The whole event was a bit of a disaster as Mike featured prominently in all my thoughts for the future. I apologised for my somewhat cool behaviour and he kindly admitted that he could see very plainly that I was still in love with Mike.

The following day, Sunday, Mike called round on the pretext of wanting to see the dogs, looking very forlorn and depressed. After a lot of coaxing I managed to drag out of him that his problem was that he really missed me and he felt he couldn't live without me.

Before I had time to think I had blurted out that I loved him too and couldn't live without him either, that I had decided not to sell the house because I just *knew* that everything was going to be all right. I explained that I had now handed my life over to the Lord who was the new 'director' of my life. That night I knew that I should marry Mike.

The week that followed was one of the happiest of my life. The joy and love in our house was overflowing. Dawn was thrilled because she got along brilliantly with Mike, and everyone else was delighted too, though my office staff must have wondered how long *this* would last after the ups and downs of our relationship during the previous few years! It was now one week to closedown.

The following Friday, Good Friday 1986, Mike and I went out for dinner to celebrate getting back together. Half way through the main course I asked him if he would be my husband. Mike nearly fainted; in fact he never did finish the meal. We were married four months later and Dawn was bridesmaid. Phil and his girlfriend Trish came to the wedding plus our relatives and a few very close friends. We had a wonderful honeymoon in Austria and have been blessed with a marvellously happy relationship ever since. Perhaps the most wonderful thing that happened to us was that a year later, Mike also become a born-again Christian, also as a result of reading *Power for Living*. That book completely changed our lives and we have never looked back. We were able to start a new life, wiping clean the slate of past living and to simply follow the path of a new life laid down for us by the Lord.

We managed to wind-up the business very satisfactorily by giving the lecturers the classes to continue in their own right. We distributed all remaining stationery so that they had a bit of a start in their new business venture and I was always available at the end of the telephone to give any help or advice. My staff in the office were very understanding when I explained that the company had to close. With the difficulties over the previous few months I think to some, closure was not totally unexpected.

Fortunately, they were all able to find alternative employment and they were able to be released as soon as they wished without it affecting their redundancy payments. I continued to handle all correspondence over the following months until all the loose ends were tidied up. Looking back, I feel the transition went quite smoothly. However, considering that I had decided to go freelance, I seemed to be working just as hard as I had previously, as now I had no secretary to type the letters or accountants to keep the books. Fortunately, Mike was around to help me and somehow we got it all done.

It was shortly after I had left Successful Slimming Clubs that I discovered the remarkable side effect of my low-fat diet – my huge hips and thighs were changing shape, right in front of my eyes! Inches of fat were disappearing from this area that had caused me constant embarrassment. The members of my classes remarked on the transformation and begged me to let them try the diet too. They enjoyed a similar benefit and after putting it to the test with a trial team the results proved its effectiveness and I realised a book had to be written. My *Hip and Thigh Diet* enjoyed even greater success than anyone had ever hoped for and I then realised why God had made me ill when he did and in fact his timing was, as always, impeccable!

Without the success of both the first *Hip and Thigh Diet* and the *Complete Hip and Thigh Diet* published earlier this year, *you* might not have bothered to buy *this* book which

17

is written by me in gratitude for all that has happened in my life. Accordingly, I am donating all royalties from this publication to charities, including the R.N.I.B. and the Leicestershire Hospice. It is my belief that we owe it to ourselves, to each other and to our maker to live life to the full, eating healthily, exercising sensibly, making the most of the beauty we have been given and adopting a positive attitude while we work, rest and play. *Looking Good Feeling Great* looks at five essential aspects of health and beauty: diet, nutrition, good grooming, exercise and positive thinking.

When life is good, looking good and feeling great will only deepen our enjoyment; when the stresses and strains of today's living knock on our doors, we will be better equipped to deal with them. It is a goal I believe we can *all* achieve.

Part 1

Slimming

What are calories?

A calorie is a unit of heat (and therefore energy). The amount of heat produced by a piece of coal is measured in calories and, similarly, our bodies burn food which produces heat or energy. Generally speaking, if we consume more calories than we burn, we store the excess in the form of fat and we gain weight. If our calorie intake equals our energy output our weight remains constant – but if we wish to reduce weight, we must eat fewer calories than we burn. That's when our bodies draw on reserve stores of fat. However, it is essential to eat sufficient of the right sort of food while dieting to remain in good health.

What is 'metabolic rate'?

Metabolism is the word used to describe the change of food into the chemical constituents the body needs to exist and grow. Metabolic rate is the rate at which one's body burns fuel or, to compare a human body with a motor car, one's rate of miles per gallon! Some people are fortunate enough to be able to eat anything and have their weight remain constant, while others seem to gain weight after eating just one good meal in a restaurant.

Overweight is a hazard of the age in which we live – motor cars, automatic washing machines, central heating and fast food all contribute to our doing less physically and the food we eat being much more readily available. Our comfortable lifestyle, with so much of the hard work done for us, means that we can gain weight very easily indeed. It almost creeps up on us without us noticing.

Being a little overweight is an inconvenience rather than a health hazard because unless we are grossly obese, our body doesn't actually suffer physically. However, the detrimental effect on our personality can be quite incredible, not to mention the embarrassment and physical discomfort experienced by those who are very overweight. One lady I knew became lodged in a turnstile as she tried to enter a football stadium. The fire brigade had to be called to release her! A friend of mine told me how a very overweight neighbour called round one day. As she plonked herself down on the sofa, there was an almighty crack and the settee sank to the floor and the arms rose heavenwards! Can you imagine the embarrassment for all concerned? Obviously overweight to this degree *is* harmful to the body. After all, our skeletons were not designed to carry such an abnormally heavy load. However, it is equally wrong to starve ourselves to achieve a skinny body which is also abnormal. Some people have little control as to their body shape and are very thin despite generous and healthy intakes of food whilst others remain quite plump eating very little.

Let's compare the person who can eat anything, yet maintains a constant weight, with a Rolls-Royce motor car. This magnificent vehicle consumes a considerable amount of petrol on a given journey compared with, say, a Mini, which will go the same distance on remarkably less fuel. Those of us who gain weight easily are, regrettably, like the Mini. When extra supplies of fuel are delivered, in effect extra fuel tanks have to be built in order to store the fuel. These stores are, in human terms, fat cells.

We cannot change the way we are made – so we must accept our 'styling' and, if we are to stop our fat stores increasing, we must stop the deliveries of fuel which are surplus to our requirements. In the short term, it is also necessary to cut back our intake in order to use up some of the accumulated stores. There is only one way to lose weight. We must consume less energy (calories) than we use. The food and drink we consume each day provides the body with energy, measured in calories.

The basal metabolic rate of an average female is approximately 1200 to 1400 calories per day – this is the number of calories she burns up in keeping her body mechanism ticking over. As soon as she starts any physical activity, she uses more fuel and therefore burns up more calories, and the more physically active she is the more calories she burns up.

A mother with three young children under school age, a husband and a home to look after, a dog to exercise regularly and no car in which to go shopping, would be classed as very active. She would probably burn in the region of 2300 to 2500 calories per day.

A mother with two school-age children, a part-time clerical job at which she sits down most of the time and a husband who dines out at lunchtime, might be classed as moderately active. She would probably burn around 2000 to 2200 calories per day.

But many women do not fall into either category and must be classed as inactive. This does not necessarily mean that they are ladies of leisure – far from it. Such a person could be a hard-working woman in a high-powered job – but most of her exertion would be in mental activity. Unfortunately, brain work doesn't burn up very many calories! Our career woman probably has her own car and, because of her lifestyle, probably doesn't have time to go shopping every day. She therefore organises herself into a weekly – or even a monthly – shopping routine. Her freezer is well stocked, her washing may be sent to the laundry and the dishwasher cleans the dishes. She may also have cleaning help in the home. Because of the very demanding nature of her work, our career woman frequently comes home in the evening feeling totally exhausted. She may watch television or read a book because she needs to relax in this way to relieve the mental stress of the office day. It is not surprising that she has little energy left for physical exercise.

A more usual 'sedentary' existence is that of the woman whose children have grown up and left home, and who has only her husband and home to care for. The rush has gone out of her life and she can take her time. As she gets older she will move about less quickly so that her calorie/energy output is inevitably lower. It is estimated that a woman in a sedentary situation burns approximately 1800 to 2000 calories per day.

It may surprise you to learn that there is a very narrow margin between each of these categories. But it must be understood that the bulk of energy/calorie output is expended in the maintenance and running of our bodies, not in the physical or mental activity they are asked to perform.

It is now accepted that exercise and activity alone are not effective ways of reducing weight – but exercise is extremely good for almost everyone and will certainly help to tone your body while you are reducing your weight. It will also promote better health.

Whether you have a metabolism like a Rolls-Royce or a Mini, you can still do something to improve your body shape if you find yourself overweight. We should look at ourselves, assess the present body state and decide whether we should be slimmer, fitter or just plain healthier. Our eating habits are very significant in achieving a fit and healthy body and if we are overweight, we must decide what is the best way to reduce our body mass.

Personally, I believe most people trying to lose weight eat far too *little* while on a slimming diet. I have found over the last seventeen years in which I have been involved in the slimming business that dieters lose at least as much, if not more, by consuming a greater number of calories than normally allowed on many slimming diets. I cannot understand why anyone starves themselves for a few days thinking that this will solve their weight problem, when they can eat good quantities of healthy low-calorie food, not feel hungry *and* lose weight at the same time! Surely this must be a more sensible solution.

What many slimmers do not understand is that our metabolic rate will adjust according to the intake of calories. If we drastically reduce our consumption of calories the body will adjust its needs so that it can survive on less food. This is why dieters often experience a 'plateau' when, despite continued dieting efforts, they do not see any further weight loss for a while – the body has adjusted its needs and manages on less. If we consider the nutritional needs of nations struck by famine it is easy to realise that the metabolic rates of the famine victims have reduced drastically. By giving them only a little food they soon respond positively and become well nourished. Reducing our metabolic rate is therefore the last thing a slimmer wants to experience. We can safeguard against such a slowing down process by consuming more calories than most diets allow yet keeping the amount below the level of calories our body needs so that we draw on our reserves of fat. This all sounds very sensible, and indeed simple, but we have to remember the lingering enemy – temptation.

Temptation is the cause of a weakening willpower. Never have the television advertisements and marketing expertise of supermarkets been so eye catching and mouth-watering. It is hard to resist such sumptuous invitations to buy! Giving in to temptation will ruin our efforts and we must endeavour to ensure that our willpower is in control of our eating and not allow the eating to control us.

Many a time I have seen others, as well as experiencing

23

it myself, feeling quite desperate about a weight problem; feeling out of control, 'possessed' almost. It completely takes over our personality and can make us quite introverted and negative. We must be aware of this situation and fight against it with confidence. Eating sensibly and not starving yourself is the only answer.

So how much can we eat and still lose weight?

Working out your daily calorie allowance

Hopefully you will now have some idea of your calorie/energy output, so we must arrive at a level of calorie intake which will effect a significant weight loss but allow you as much food as possible to avoid getting hungry. If you enjoy your diet and never feel hungry, your chances of keeping to it are considerably greater!

When you embark on a reducing diet, the area of your body is at its greatest. As it reduces in size, it obviously requires less fuel to maintain it. So after shedding a stone (6 kilos) or so, your body may not reduce its weight on the calorie allowance with which you started your slimming campaign. Should you wish to reduce your weight further, a reduction in your daily calorie intake of approximately 100–200 would soon effect acceptable weight losses again. Continue on this lower calorie intake until your body reaches another plateau after losing another 1.5 to 2 stones (8.5–12.5 kilos), then again reduce your daily allowance.

In my experience I have found that slimmers reach a plateau whether they start on 1000 calories a day or 1600 calories a day. The poor 1000-a-day slimmer is going to feel ravenous on the 700 calories to which she may find she has to reduce in order to shift those last few pounds (or kilos). On the other hand, with my method of maximum calories, no one need ever fall below a daily intake of 1000 calories. In fact, I would definitely advise that they should not!

The following table illustrates the ideal calorie intake

	Estimated energy/ calorie output	Initial calorie allowance	Reducing calorie allowances		
			1st	2nd	Final
Women					
Very active	2500	1700	1500	1400	1200
Active	2200	1600	1400	1250	1100
Moderately active	2000	1500	1300	1150	1050
Sedentary	1800 2000	1400	1200	1100	1000
Men					
Very active	3500 4000	2500	2200	2000	1800
Active	3000 3350	2100	1950	1750	1650
Moderately active	2700	1900	1800	1650	1550
Sedentary	2500	1800	1700	1600	1500

Anyone who is grossly overweight should increase the above allowances as follows:

Stones (kilos) overweight	Extra daily calorie allowance
3 (19)	50
4 (25.5)	100
5 (32)	150
6 (38)	200
7 (44.5)	250
8 (51)	300
9 (57)	350
10 (63.5)	400

according to your activity rating – and keep to the maximum calorie allowance for as long as possible. Only reduce your calorie intake if no weight loss has occurred for at least two weeks. Always take the next lower rating; never try to take short cuts to an even lower calorie allowance.

Slimming on the maximum number of calories

Remember, it is advisable to consult your doctor before embarking on a reducing diet – particularly if you have in excess of a stone (6 kilos) to lose. But argue if he says you should stick to 1000 calories per day. I promise you that ninety-nine people out of every hundred who are overweight will lose weight more effectively on a considerably higher intake and are far less likely to regain their lost weight yet keeping the amount below the level of calories our body needs so that we draw on our reserves of fat.

It is reasonable to assume that if each of us looks different on the outside we must also vary on the inside. Consequently our needs for food and nourishment must vary from one person to another. However, if we are overweight we must have some idea whether we got that way by being a nibbler, a sipper or a plain straightforward gannet! Overweight is almost definitely caused by consuming too many calories. Only one in a million can blame obesity on glands or illness.

The no-calorie counting alternative

Some people are quite slim except in certain areas, in fact they could be simply categorised as having a busty, hippy or roly-poly figure type. For these slimmers it could be more beneficial to follow a very low-fat diet such as my Hip and Thigh Diet, which whilst sounding only suitable for pear shaped people, it does in fact work in correcting figure faults generally.

The basis of this diet is not calorie counting but very low fat content. Weight for weight fat has twice the calorie content of carbohydrate so if you can cut the fat to a minimum you automatically cut out a great number of calories. You can then eat great quantities of carbohydrate foods plus some low fat proteins and still lose weight.

There have been extensive studies in nutritional laboratories which have produced convincing evidence that those following a diet high in carbohydrate weigh less than those consuming a high fat diet containing the same number of calories. The conclusion reached is that the body utilises carbohydrate calories much more efficiently than fat calories because carbohydrate calories burn clean.

So why are fats so bad? First of all, a diet high in fat can seriously affect our health. It can raise the level of cholesterol and uric acid in our body tissue. It can also hinder the body metabolism of carbohydrate and encourage diabetes. But perhaps most important of all, fat forms a film around the formed elements of the blood, in particular the red blood cells and platelets causing them to stick together and this obviously leads to less efficient functioning with some small blood vessels and capillaries becoming shut down altogether. This means that about 10 per cent of our blood circulation is shut down. And don't be fooled into thinking that saturated fats are worse than polyunsaturated fats – they're all as bad as each other and anyone who suffers with a high cholesterol problem should reduce *all* fats.

We are told by manufacturers of polyunsaturated margarines that their products will lower cholesterol levels. This is true but they omit to point out that they may significantly increase the levels of triglycerides creating metabolic suffocation by the resulting sludge in the blood.

Also, vital for the slimmer to know, is that margarines low in cholesterol (polyunsaturates) are most definitely *not* lower in calories. And don't think they are lower in fat either. The fat content is exactly the same. The only substitutes that *can* help the slimmer are those that state they are 'low-fat' e.g. Gold, Outline etc. Earlier this year a new product called 'Gold Lowest' was launched and this contains a quarter of the fat and calories of all butters and margarines.

However, whilst following the Hip and Thigh Diet no butter or butter alternatives are allowed nor fatty products such as chocolate, biscuits, cakes, crisps, chips or nuts.

The good news though is that this diet achieves the most incredible results as anyone who has followed it will tell you. Instead of losing inches from the parts of your body you wish to keep, slimmers lose inches from their outsized areas. Never has a diet achieved such amazing results in reshaping the human body. It works equally well for men too but on their tums not their thighs (men don't suffer with big thighs but usually store their fat on their stomach).

This diet is extensively explained in my books *Hip and Thigh Diet* and *The Complete Hip and Thigh Diet*. However, in *this* book I offer a suggested menu following the rules of *The Complete Hip and Thigh Diet*, along with an assortment of other menus from which you may choose to suit your individual taste and circumstances. You may find a very low fat diet too restricting but on the other hand many have written to me saying it isn't like a diet at all! The important thing is for you to find a diet or way of eating that suits *you*.

When you have achieved your weight goal and are managing to keep your weight reasonably stable by eating sensibly, you will be able to enjoy a more relaxed attitude towards your food and fluid intake. This will make life much more enjoyable and you will gain more confidence in your ability to control your eating habits. The panic experienced by dieters who go 'off the rails' soon disappears.

Your ideal weight

You will not find an 'ideal weight' chart in this book as I do not believe in them. *You* know whether or not you are overweight just by looking at yourself in the mirror with no clothes on! Recommended weights can vary so much according to bone structure that few people are able to calculate accurately their own 'ideal' weight. They often add a little to their height to take them into the next weight bracket and then feel delighted to read that their weight is said to be 'ideal'! But the midriff bulge is still there and so are the heavy, bulging thighs.

Your ideal weight is the weight at which you look your most attractive, though this may be half a stone (3 kilos) heavier or lighter than is recommended by the charts.

Speed of weight loss

Before embarking on any form of reducing diet, you must realise that to lose weight your body must burn up some of its reserves which are stored in the form of fat. There is obviously a limit to how fast this can be done and you must accept the fact that a certain amount of patience is needed for you to reach your desired weight.

Crash diets are a complete waste of time and I do not propose to waste space discussing them except to point out that they can be damaging to health as they can cause a reduction in muscle tissue as well as fat. However, an occasional one-day fast or a very low-calorie day following an over-eating spell can prove to be invaluable.

I am always being asked how quickly people can lose weight on my diets. I can only say that different people react in different ways on different diets – but if the suggested diets are adhered to totally, weight loss can be considerable.

Occasionally, quite early on in your dieting campaign, you may find that your weight remains constant even though you have been particularly strict with yourself. This is a peculiarity of the human body and is completely beyond our control. If you have not adhered to your present calorie allowance for very long, please do not reduce it further as it may not be the calorie intake that has produced the plateau, but possibly fluid level variation. Continue with your diet regardless, taking particular care to count every mouthful. Soon your body will regulate itself once more and you will again see a reduction in your weight.

Many women find that a significant weight gain occurs just prior to a menstrual period – an increase of as much as six pounds (2.75 kilos) is not unusual. However, some women experience no such increase at this time but at some other time during their menstrual cycle, at a regular time each month. Also many women find dieting difficult prior to menstruation as they often feel very low or depressed. If you suffer in this way, it would be sensible to anticipate a possible lack of willpower at this time and so allow a more generous diet, trying also to busy yourself with some hobby that you enjoy.

What makes a good diet?

A good diet is a diet which is successful. For it to be successful:

1 It must be nutritionally sound.
2 It must appeal to you.
3 It must fit into your lifestyle.
4 There must be a margin of freedom.
5 It must contain enough food to prevent you from feeling hungry.
6 It must be flexible so that dining out can be enjoyable.
7 It should contain everyday foods and avoid additional expense.
8 It should be adaptable so that the rest of the family may be fed on similar food.

9 It should contain plenty of variety.
10 It should contain foods that you enjoy eating.

You may feel that this list of requirements would be impossible to find – but I assure you that it is possible to find the perfect diet for you.

On the pages that follow you will find a variety of diets. They have all been exhaustively tested for their effectiveness. They have also all been examined and found to be nutritionally sound in their composition.

The following Hip and Thigh Diet does not involve any calorie counting because it automatically cuts out a great number of calories by the elimination of all visible fats. Further, by greatly reducing those foods which do contain fat it enables us to enjoy considerable freedom of choice of those foods which contain little or no fat.

Diet 1: The Hip and Thigh Diet

Methods of Preparation and Notes.

Grill, boil, bake or microwave – never fry.
Remove all visible fat and skin before cooking.
Unlimited vegetables means just that. No need to weigh these items but they must be cooked without fat.
All bread should be wholemeal when possible.
1 piece of fruit = 1 apple or orange or 1 slice of pineapple
(1 piece = 4 – 5 oz)

Diet Rules

Try not to eat between meals. Menu suggestions can be changed around to suit your individual taste but do stick to the principle of three meals – a breakfast, lunch and dinner menu. If you wish you may take a multi-vitamin tablet daily though I do not consider this to be necessary if you eat the selection of foods I have suggested.

Don't cheat. This diet will only work effectively if you strictly follow the 'very low fat' ruling.

HIP AND THIGH DIET

Daily allowance: ½ pint (10fl oz) skimmed or semi-skimmed milk, 2 alcoholic drinks e.g. 2 glasses wine, 2 single measures of any spirit served with low calorie mixers.

	Monday	Tuesday	Wednesday	Thursday	Friday	Saturday	Sunday
Breakfast	1oz Porridge made with water and served with milk from allowance and 2 tsps honey	1oz Branflakes with milk from allowance and 1 tsp sugar	4–5 pieces of fresh fruit	½ fresh grapefruit. 1 slice toast with 2 tsps of marmalade	5 prunes in natural juice, plus 5oz plain low-fat yoghurt	6oz baked beans on slice toast	1oz very lean bacon, 2 fresh tomatoes, grilled or small tin of tomatoes. 1 slice toast
Lunch	4–5 pieces of any fresh fruit (e.g. 1 orange = 1 fruit)	4 slices 'light' bread or 3oz ordinary wholemeal bread, made into sandwiches with 1oz chicken and unlimited salad vegetables plus 2 tsps Branston Pickle	4 Ryvitas spread with 2 tsps Branston Pickle plus 4 slices of chicken 'roll' or 3oz chicken or turkey breast. 2 tomatoes. Diet yoghurt	Large salad plus 2oz lean ham or 3oz chicken plus 1tbsp reduced oil dressing e.g. Waistline	Jacket potato (5–10oz) topped with cottage cheese (4oz) and chopped onion	3oz pilchards or salmon with large salad and oil-free vinaigrette dressing. Diet yoghurt	6oz chicken (no skin) or 3oz beef – (no fat) served with unlimited vegetables and thin gravy. Stuffed apple and plain yoghurt.
Dinner	Wedge of melon. 6oz chicken, all skin removed, with unlimited vegetables including potatoes. Served with a little thin gravy. Diet yoghurt	½ Grapefruit. 3oz very lean pork or lamb with unlimited vegetables. Served with a little thin gravy. Sliced banana topped with diet yoghurt	Clear soup. 8oz fish (white) served with unlimited vegetables and tomato sauce if desired. Fresh fruit salad	Ratatouille. Vegetable bake. Stuffed apple with plain yoghurt.	Orange and grape-fruit cocktail. Fish pie (see recipe). Raspberries in a meringue basket topped with rasp-berry yoghurt or fromage frais	Garlic mushrooms. 4oz steak or 6oz liver, served with unlimited vegetables and jacket potato. Pears in red wine	French tomatoes Cottage cheese salad. Wedge of melon

The Forbidden List

Butter, margarine and all low fat and low cholesterol products (e.g. Outline, Gold, Flora etc).
All cream and cream alternatives, Coffeemate, whole milk, gold top milk.
Lard, oil (all kinds) dripping, suet etc.
Milk puddings and milk products.
Fried foods of any kind.
Fat or skin from meat, poultry or game.
Egg yolks (egg whites may be eaten).
Fatty fish including mackerel, kippers, rollmop herrings, eels, herrings, sardines, bloaters, tuna, sprats and whitebait.
All nuts except chestnuts.
Sunflower seeds.
Goose.
All fatty meats e.g. salami, sausages, pate.
Avocados, chocolates, fudge, toffees, lemon curd.
Sauces and puddings made with fat.
Cakes, pastry, biscuits, crispbreads (except Ryvita).

Fish Pie
(Serves 4)

1½ lbs (700 g) cod
1½ lbs (700 g) potatoes
salt and pepper

Bake, steam or microwave the fish but do not overcook. Season well.

Boil the potatoes until well done and mash with a little water to make a soft consistency. Season well.

Place fish in an ovenproof dish. Flake the flesh, remove the skin, and distribute the fish evenly across the base of the dish.

Cover the fish completely with the mashed potatoes and smooth over with a fork.

If the ingredients are still hot just place under a hot grill for a few minutes to brown the top. Alternatively the pie can be made well in advance and then warmed through in a preheated moderate oven (180°C, 350°F, Gas Mark 4) for 20 minutes, or microwaved on *high* for 5 minutes.

Note to Vegetarians

On the Hip and Thigh Diet vegetarians may include the following foods instead of meat, fish and poultry, prepared in the normal way without any fat.

4 oz: Black eyed beans
Butter beans
Chick peas
Continental lentils
Green split peas
Haricot beans
Lentils
Red kidney beans
Yellow split peas

An egg may be eaten in exchange for a 4–6 oz meat portion, but do not eat more than three in a week. This is allowable for vegetarians because they eat most of their protein in lentils and pulses which are very low in fat content. An occasional egg, whilst quite high in fat, should not therefore jeopardise the diet for vegetarians.

I accept that not everyone wishes to follow a very low fat diet even though I believe it is the healthiest way of eating. The following two diets are the ones that have been used at my slimming clubs during the past seventeen years. They are very effective in achieving an excellent weight loss and have proved very popular with slimmers.

The calorie content of Diet 2 is around 1400 calories a day. Don't forget to eat the greater number of calories when you first start dieting, and reduce to 1200 later, when

you are slimmer. Don't try to cut corners and go without –
dieting doesn't work that way. Our bodies need a constant
supply of necessary nutrients to operate healthily and
efficiently.

Diet 2: 1400 Calorie Diet

Notes

Drinks may be taken freely between meals using milk from
the allowance. 'Slimline' or 'Diet' low-calorie drinks may
be taken freely.
Weights quoted are cooked weights.
Your 100 calorie 'treat allowance' may be used daily or
saved up for a special occasion each week, but don't expect
to weigh less the day after you have consumed the lot at
one sitting! It is better to split up your treats over several
days.
   Do eat what is recommended. Don't cut foods out
thinking you will lose more weight. It doesn't work like
that. All that happens is that you will double your chances
of giving in to temptation and having a binge.

Diet 3: 1200 Calorie Diet

This is another calorie-counted diet offering a wide variety
of everyday foods but the style of this diet offers maximum
freedom of choice and versatility.
   You are allowed three meals a day – one from each
category, plus a treat of your choice totalling no more than
150 calories. The meals and the treat can be eaten any time.
Of course, if you prefer this diet to the previous 1400 calorie
diet, you can increase the quantities of the portions or add
extra potatoes or fruit to make up to a total 1400 a day.
The choice is yours.

DIET 2 - Approximately 1400 calories per day

Daily allowance: ½ pint whole milk, ¼ oz low fat spread, preferably Gold Lowest.

	Monday	Tuesday	Wednesday	Thursday	Friday	Saturday	Sunday
Breakfast	1 scrambled egg 1oz wholemeal toast 2 tomatoes	½ grapefruit 1oz grilled bacon 1 fried egg cooked in very litte fat ½ oz wholemeal bread	½ grapefruit 1 boiled egg 1oz wholemeal bread	1 small carton plain yoghurt, 1 teaspoon honey plus 1 teaspoon chopped nuts	Small glass of unsweetened fruit juice. 1oz grilled bacon 2 tomatoes grilled ½ oz wholemeal toast	1 piece fresh fruit 1oz grilled bacon 2 tomatoes grilled	½ grapefruit 1oz wholemeal toast 2 teaspoons marmalade
Lunch	1 cup-a-soup (8oz) Large salad with 2oz ham	Large salad with 4oz cottage cheese or 1oz hard cheese plus 1oz Waistline or similar dressing 1 pear	2 slices wholemeal bread, spread with Waistline dressing and filled with 1oz ham and salad 1 apple	2 slices wholemeal bread, spread with Waistline dressing and filled with 1oz hard cheese and salad 1 orange	3oz tinned mackerel, plus large mixed salad. 1 tbsp of Waistline dressing. 2oz grapes.	2 beefburgers 1 tomato 2oz mushrooms 4oz vegetables 2oz chips. Diet yoghurt	4oz roast meat 6oz green veg 1 jacket potato (2oz) Thin gravy 4oz fresh fruit salad.
Dinner	4oz lean meat or offal 2oz jacket or boiled potato 8oz green vegetables Little gravy 4oz fresh fruit salad	6oz grilled plaice or cod 8oz green vegetables 4oz carrots 2oz chips Diet yoghurt	½ pint clear soup 1 grilled lean lamb chop 2oz jacket or boiled potato 4oz carrots 4oz cauliflower or cabbage Diet yoghurt	4 fish fingers, grilled 3oz peas 4oz carrots 2oz chips 1 tablespoon tomato ketchup, if desired 2oz grapes	4oz chicken 2oz jacket potato 4oz cabbage 4oz green beans 4oz carrots Thin gravy. 1 orange.	3oz ham and salad with Waistline dressing Fresh fruit salad	Cottage cheese (4oz) on 4 crispbreads Tomato and cucumber Diet yoghurt and a piece of fruit.
	PLUS: 100 Calorie Treat	PLUS: 100 Calorie Treat	PLUS: 100 Calorie Treat	PLUS: 100 Calorie Treat	PLUS: 100 Calorie Treat	PLUS: 100 Calorie Treat	PLUS: 100 Calorie Treat

Diet 3

To be consumed daily

300ml: ½ pint fresh milk or 600ml: 1 pint skimmed milk
15g: ½ oz low-fat spread
Tea and coffee may be drunk freely, provided that your
milk allowance is not exceeded and that artificial sweeteners
are used in place of sugar. Low-calorie squashes, slimline
drinks, pure lemon juice and water are also unrestricted.

Breakfasts

1   ½ fresh grapefruit, 1 boiled or poached egg, 25g/1oz
    bread, butter from allowance.
2   ½ fresh grapefruit, 25g/1oz grilled lean bacon,
    100g/4oz tomatoes, 25g/1oz bread, 15g/½oz
    marmalade, low fat spread from allowance.
3   90ml/3fl oz unsweetened orange juice, 15g/½oz
    cornflakes or similar cereal, 150ml/¼ pint milk
    (additional to allowance) 1 teaspoon sugar.
4   ½ fresh grapefruit, 1 Weetabix or Shredded Wheat or
    3 tablespoons All Bran, 150ml/¼ pint milk (additional
    to allowance), 2 teaspoons sugar.

Main meals

1   175ml/6oz clear or low calorie soup. 75g/3oz lean red
    meat or 100g/4oz chicken or 225g/8oz steamed white
    fish, 100g/4oz green leafy vegetables, 100g/4oz carrots,
    50g/2oz potato (new or jacket), little thin gravy (Oxo
    or similar) if desired. 100g/4oz stewed fruit (no sugar).
2   Large salad comprising lettuce, tomatoes, cucumber,
    celery, spring onions, grated raw carrot, ½ hard-boiled
    egg, and 50g/2oz cold lean meat or 75g/3oz chicken
    or 25g/1oz hard cheese (e.g. Cheddar) or 100g/4oz
    cottage cheese. 25g/1oz low-calorie salad dressing.
    75g/3oz jacket potato or 25g/1oz bread (butter from

allowance). 100g/4oz stewed fruit (no sugar) or baked apple.

3   175ml/6fl oz clear or low calorie soup. 50g/2oz liver, 25g/1oz grilled lean bacon, 2 tomatoes, 50g/2oz thick-cut chips, 100g/4oz green beans. 100g/4oz fresh fruit salad. 1 large sausage, 1 fried egg, 50g/2oz thick-cut chips, 2 grilled tomatoes, 100g/4oz green leafy vegetables, 100g/4oz carrots. 25g/1oz ice-cream.

4   Two egg omelette with 15g/½oz hard cheese and 50g/2oz grilled mushrooms, large salad, 100g/4oz jacket potato or 50g/2oz thick cut chips, 1 small pear.

Snack Meals

1   25g/1oz toast with 15g/½oz hard cheese and one poached egg, garnished with 1 sliced tomato.

2   50g/2oz bread made into a sandwich with lettuce, cucumber, tomato, 2 slices hard-boiled egg, 15g/½oz grated cheese. Use a little low-calorie salad dressing if desired.

3   1 fried egg, 50g/2oz thick-cut chips, 50g/2oz peas.

4   2 cream crackers or crispbreads 15g/½oz hard cheese, 150g/5oz carton fruit yoghurt or 2 pieces fresh fruit.

5   100g/4oz ham or 2 hard-boiled eggs with salad, 1 crispbread.

6   100g/4oz cottage cheese (with or without chives or pineapple) on two crispbreads.

7   1 small tin of one of the following: spaghetti bolognaise, spaghetti in tomato and cheese sauce, spaghetti hoops, ravioli or baked beans, plus 25g/1oz toast.

You may have one 'treat' per day amounting to approximately 150 calories. A few suggestions are as follows:

small packet of crisps
3 diet yoghurts
extra 300ml/½ pint fresh milk
2 tablespoons double cream

25g/1oz sweets
1 doughnut
65g/2½oz ice-cream
1 small cake
2 chocolate digestive biscuits
300ml/½ pint beer
2 pub measures of any spirit
25g/1oz of chocolate
3 plain biscuits

In fact, you may choose anything providing the calorie value does not exceed 150. If in doubt as to the calorie values buy a calorie book from your local bookshop.

Ten tips for successful slimming

1 Substitute artificial sweeteners for sugar in tea, coffee and cooking.
2 Always grill, boil, steam, dry-roast or microwave food rather than fry it.
3 Don't go shopping when you feel hungry because you're likely to gorge yourself when you get home.
4 If there's a particular food you can't resist – don't have it in the home.
5 When dining out, don't start drinking alcohol until you've started the main course. Your willpower will weaken with the alcohol.
6 Keep some diet drinks in the fridge so that whenever you feel really hungry you can drink one to help fill you up before you eat too much.
7 At that time of the month when your willpower may be weak or you have a craving for something sweet, keep lots of low-calorie, low-fat yoghurts in the fridge to treat yourself. Diet Coke is a great sweet-tooth soother too.
8 Stop making excuses for cheating. If you're going to eat something you shouldn't, own up – don't kid yourself that an excuse makes it all right! Also

WEIGHT LOSS AND INCH LOSS RECORD

DATE:																	
Weight																	
Total weight lost to date																	
Bust																	
Waist																	
Hips																	
Widest part																	
L. Thigh																	
R. Thigh																	
L. Knee																	
R. Knee																	
L. Arm																	
R. Arm																	
Total inches this week																	
Total to date																	

remember that one cheat won't ruin the diet. And if you continue cheating because you feel you've 'blown it', you will undo all the good work.

9 Try to increase your energy output while you are slimming. This is the *only* way you can make your diet work faster. Cutting extra calories won't speed up your weight loss but increasing your calorie output will.

10 Buy a tape measure and measure your progress weekly as well as monitoring your weight loss on the scales. Better still, get your husband or someone to do it for you.

Part 2

Nutrition

Basic nutrition

Food contains five types of nutrients.
Proteins which help to build body cells and supply energy.
Carbohydrates and *Fats* which supply energy (alcohol falls into this category)
Minerals which help to build some parts of the body, protect it from deficiency diseases and regulate metabolism.
Vitamins which help to regulate metabolism, fight infection and also protect the body from deficiency diseases.

Proteins

Foods high in protein are cheese, eggs, meat, fish, poultry, game, pulses, soya flour, wholemeal flour and nuts. We used to be told that we need a lot of protein in our daily diet but recent investigations have proved that too much protein in fact can be harmful to our health.

We do of course need some protein but it is protein's components – the amino acids – which are essential for life. As protein is digested it is broken down into these organic acids which play an important role in growth, metabolism and the repair and maintenance of our body tissues. There are twenty-two amino acids of which fourteen can be manufactured by the body. The remainder are only available from food.

Another misapprehension is that these foods listed above are the *only* sources of protein. Nothing could be further from the truth! Almost all foods contain protein and often in surprisingly large amounts. For instance ounce for ounce, there is as much protein in wholewheat cereal or porridge as there is in eggs. Fruit and vegetables, crisps and snacks, biscuits and crispbreads, rice and pasta – they all contain protein. So there is no danger whatever of becoming deficient in protein in this country where food is plentiful.

I am not suggesting we should cut out the foods high in protein (meat, fish, eggs and cheese) but we should eat them in moderation, not excess. If you are following a very low fat diet take your protein in white fish, poultry, cottage cheese and wholewheat cereals and baked beans as well as in fruit and vegetables.

Carbohydrates

Carbohydrates give us energy and are burned very efficiently by the body. Only carbohydrates burn 100 per cent clean – converting into energy, carbon dioxide (which is breathed out) and water (which is excreted in urine, faeces and perspiration). The more 'complete' or unrefined the carbohydrate, the better it is, e.g., wholegrain cereals and grains, fruits and vegetables. Refined carbohydrates such as sugar are not good and should be keep to a minimum.

Endurance athletes consume vast quantities of carbohydrates, not protein, to give them strength and stamina. It is unfortunate that carbohydrates have been given a bad name in the past with favour being given to proteins. With the advancement in medical investigation of the effect food has on our health, the tide now has turned. Evidence supports the theory that a diet high in protein can cause heart disease, whereas a diet high in carbohydrate is extremely healthy.

Fats

The main purpose of fat is that it provides energy (calories) which is fine if you are underweight, but an enemy to the slimmer.

We can get all the energy we need from carbohydrates and proteins so additional fat in our diet is quite unnecessary. It is impossible to eat no fat as most foods contain some – the secret is to consume foods with a lower fat content whenever possible.

Our bodies need a certain amount of fat but can manufacture almost all the fats they need from other foods. If you eat a varied diet including unrefined grains such as wholemeal bread, cereals and oats, there is no risk of deficiency.

From the amazing success in reducing inches not touched by other diets by slimmers who followed my Hip and Thigh Diet, it is obvious that fat, if eaten in excess, is deposited on the body. If a big reduction in fat intake is made, these inches burn away. They will not be replaced until extra fat is reintroduced into the daily diet.

Minerals

Minerals such as calcium and iron are essential to health and provided we eat a varied and balanced diet there is little risk of deficiency.

The time to be cautious is if you eliminate from your diet one particular range of products. Skimmed or semi-skimmed milk, for instance, is a rich form of calcium, but if you drink only black tea and coffee, eat no cheese or milk products – you are likely to become deficient in calcium – the mineral needed for healthy bones and teeth. Calcium is added to bread and flour and is found in dark green vegetables but you would need to eat a great deal of these foods to consume an adequate quantity. In this case it would be wise to consult your doctor and he may suggest you take a calcium supplement.

Iron, on the other hand, is needed particularly by women as it is the nutrient required to make haemoglobin of blood and a deficiency would cause anaemia. Women lose blood during menstruation so it is most important that their diet contains an adequate ration of iron. Foods rich in iron are liver and kidney, red meat and eggs, and to a lesser degree poultry, fish, peas, bread and yoghurt.

Women are usually given an iron supplement during pregnancy because of the needs of the unborn child.

Other minerals are potassium, copper, and iodine. Potassium helps to keep our skin healthy looking and is necessary for normal growth. It stimulates the nerve impulses for muscle contraction and can be found in milk, citrus fruits, bananas, green peppers, green vegetables, tomatoes and dried fruit. Copper is involved in the storage of iron for haemoglobin formation for red blood cells. It is necessary for proper blood cell production. Copper is to be found in green vegetables. Iodine is involved in the thyroid gland secretion of thyroxine, that regulates metabolism and energy. It also affects growth and hormone production. Traces of iodine can be found in common salt and kelp.

Vitamins

There are two types of vitamins: water-soluble and fat-soluble. Water-soluble vitamins must be consumed daily as they cannot be stored in the body, whereas fat-soluble vitamins can be stored, so daily consumption is not essential. Vitamin A is a fat-soluble vitamin which helps to give a healthy skin and helps our eyesight. It is found in margarine, liver, cod liver oil, cheese, butter, eggs, kidneys, chicken, milk, carrots, spinach, watercress, tomatoes and fruits.

B vitamins are water soluble. The B complex is a group of thirteen chemically unrelated substances. Basically vitamin B is necessary to the nervous system and should never be neglected. It is found in wholegrains, yoghurt, leafy green vegetables, lean meat, Marmite, liver, cheese, eggs, milk, oatmeal, soya, peas and cereal. Wholemeal bread is a rich source of vitamin B and should be chosen in preference to white bread, though these days white bread does have added vitamins.

Vitamin C is also water-soluble. It helps us to resist infection and is found in fresh and frozen fruit and vegetables, especially citrus fruits, fruit juices, tomatoes and green vegetables. However, vitamin C is easily destroyed by overcooking, keeping food warm or by adding bicarbonate of soda during cooking. Storing fresh vegetables for several days also causes loss of vitamin content. It is also therefore a good idea to eat plenty of raw vegetables whenever possible and to shop regularly to ensure adequate supplies.

Vitamin D is also a fat-soluble vitamin and it works with calcium in the formation of healthy bones and teeth. Vitamin D is found in margarine, eggs, milk (particularly evaporated), fatty fish such as tuna, salmon and cod liver oil. We can also take in vitamin D from the sun: the sun rays fall on the skin and convert a substance in our bodies into vitamin D.

Vitamin E is a fat-soluble vitamin necessary to protect you from the dangers of oils. When we eat polyunsaturated oils we run the risk of creating quite a severe oxidising condition. Research has shown that this kind of liquid peroxidation can apparently poison the body and accelerate ageing. That is why we are told by the advertisers to take vitamin E to stay younger looking. But of course if we reduce the fat in our diet in the first place we don't need so much vitamin E to resolve the problem. The answer therefore, must be to reduce our fat intake and enjoy the benefits of a youthful skin. To prove the point further, over 35 per cent of my trial team who followed my very low fat Hip and Thigh Diet said their skin had improved. A varied diet should include wholegrain cereals, wheatgerm, lettuce, apples, carrots and cabbage.

Vitamin K, a water-soluble vitamin, is essential for normal blood clotting. It can be found in leafy green vegetables, eggs, oats, potatoes and wheatgerm, and if you consume a varied diet, there is little fear of a deficiency.

Part 3

Looking Good

In the following pages I give basic principles for making the most of hair, make-up, how to look after your skin, how to dress to flatter your figure and minimise your figure faults and how to generally present yourself to the world in the most attractive way possible.

I think it is important to realise that we can learn a great deal simply by looking around us. In fact our best guide to colours is to just look at nature and to see the colours that are blended together and which work so beautifully enhancing one another. We are able to 'come alive' in the reflection of certain colours, whereas the wrong shades can make us look washed-out and lifeless. Strangely few people realise how important correct colouring can be.

There are several organisations which offer a service called 'Colour Coding' or 'Colour Analysis' and they offer you a thorough consulation to discuss your individual colouring. Samples of fabrics are draped next to your face so that you can instantly see which colours warm towards you and which ones make you look dull and lifeless. This service is quite expensive, but I personally feel that it can be very worthwhile in avoiding those awful mistakes that we have all made in the past when we have bought a wonderful new outfit that we feel is going to steal the show, only to realise when we wear it it doesn't look quite as good as it should. We are told by these consultants that our colouring is based on a season, and people who are Winter can wear the more bold colours like bright red, black and white – the colours normally associated with Winter, whereas those with Summer colouring would wear pinky blues and bright pastel shades. Autumn colouring commands oranges, browns and creams, whereas Spring brings forth thoughts of yellows and pastel greens. If you are interested in extending your knowledge of these seasons it could be well worthwhile arranging to see your local Colour Consultant.

Everyone of us is an individual and it is important to develop our own personal style. Often we look to others for inspiration when we are not quite sure what we would like. This is particularly obvious in children approaching teenage who all copy one another at school not knowing in quite which direction to go. As we get older we prefer to develop our own individuality and, in fact, take it as a compliment if anyone copies one of our ideas. But if we are going to look our best all the while, we have to look at ourselves very impartially and decide which are our good points and which are our bad, which points we want to highlight and which aspects we want to camouflage. With this in mind I will now go through every aspect of grooming.

Hair

There is no better way to change your image and to feel better about yourself than to have a new hairstyle.

Everyone is an individual and face shapes can vary quite considerably due to the arrangement of bone structure, muscle tissue and skin. As the hair is so close to the face it can (and indeed should) be used as one would use make-up – to accentuate the good points and detract from the poor ones. Before you walk into your favourite salon with a copy of a magazine illustrating models or a movie star showing their crowning glory, ask yourself if your hair is capable of such a style. No hairdresser can easily change naturally curly hair, for instance, into a straight and flowing style. Similarly a thin head of hair would never produce a long thick curly style. Your stylist can advise you on the best style to suit your hair and your face shape, but here are some basic guidelines.

The ideal face is oval with prominent cheekbones, and a hairstyle should be designed with this in mind.

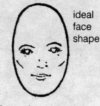

ideal face shape

Figure 1

A round face needs height in the hairstyle, but no width. There should not be a heavy fringe.

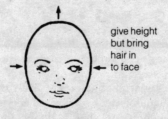

give height but bring hair in to face

Figure 2

A long face needs width and not height. Hair should be no longer than jaw level, and some hair should cover part of the forehead. Do not have a centre parting.

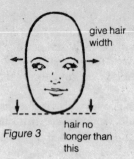

give hair
width

Figure 3

hair no
longer than
this

A face with a heavy or square jaw needs lift or width between the eyes. Hair around the jaw will only emphasise the squareness.

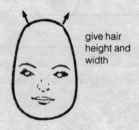

give hair
height and
width

Figure 4

As a general rule the higher the parting the longer the face appears. The fuller the fringe, the wider the face appears.

The two important qualities of lovely hair are condition and cut. Condition can be improved effectively and quickly by using a conditioner that is suitable for your hair type, for instance, for dry or oily hair. A good, healthy diet is also important. Too much heat or chemical treatments will damage the hair to the point of splitting or breaking. Split ends can only be cured by being cut off. If you become unwell at any time this will have a detrimental effect on the behaviour of your hair, too. Although it is necessary to have professional treatment for cutting and other technical services, most of us can deal with our hair at home between visits to the hairdresser. Depending on the way the hair is handled, much unnecessary damage can be caused, so think about prevention rather than cure.

Take note of the following points:

Do not use excessive heat – curling tongs, hot brushes or heated rollers should not be used too often. A blow-air brush is much kinder to the hair. Do not hold your hair dryer too close, or expose hair to strong sunlight or even ultraviolet light.

Do not use damaging tools – metal combs, rough-edged plastic combs or extra-hard nylon brushes.

Do not grip or pin the hair constantly in the same place – rubber bands are particularly damaging.

Do not pull hair tangles when the hair is wet.

Do use conditioners to lubricate the ends.

Do use good-quality combs and brushes.

Do cover the hair when you are in extreme weather conditions (e.g. strong sunlight, blustery winds).

Remember that shampooing plays a large part in the conditioning process.

The following ideas can combine to make the correct formula for the individual:

Oily hair (and scalp) needs washing every two to four days. Use a liquid shampoo, one application only. It is a good idea to dilute the shampoo first. Always use tepid, not hot, water and do not massage the scalp. Instead rub lightly with the flat of the hand.

Dry hair (and scalp) needs washing every six to eight days. Use a cream shampoo, one application only. Try to create a lather before applying and use warm water to stimulate the scalp. Massage the scalp thoroughly with your finger tips and rinse carefully. Use conditioning creams whenever possible.

Normal hair (and scalp) needs washing every four to six days. Use a variation between dry and oily treatment.

Combination hair that is oily at the roots and dry at the ends (usually long hair) is generally better treated as if dry hair, otherwise the ends become overwashed and 'fly away'. After a while it may become necessary to change the 'formula', or product used, as the scalp can become immune to the action of just one.

Colouring and permanent-wave products are now more readily available for home use. If these are going to be used it must be remembered that they are chemicals, some quite harmful, and should be treated with care. Approximately 80 per cent of heads of hair in poor condition are due to incorrect home-colouring and permanent waving. For colouring, the important rule to remember is that semi-permanent colour will *not* lighten hair at all, and will wash out after about six shampoos. When hair is lightened, even half a shade, this is permanent and the hair will not return to its natural colour except in new growth. If there are any doubts at all, seek advice from a reputable hairdresser.

You should bear in mind that if your hairstyle is to change, the following order of events should be followed:

Improve the condition first.
Visit your hairdresser for a professional cut or restyle – this is **essential**.
If your hair is in good condition then colouring could be undertaken.
If your hair has taken the colour treatment without losing any condition, permanent waving could also be undertaken.

Skin Care

I believe it was a famous gentleman who said on his eighty-sixth birthday, 'If I'd known I was going to live this long

I'd have taken better care of myself.' So often we make excuses for not taking extra effort to help us stay youthful. 'My mother and grandmother only used soap and water and they had beautiful skin' is a common remark made by those reluctant to use skin care products such as creams, milks and lotions.

Prior to 1950 few had the luxury of central heating which is very drying to the skin. We compound the problem now by going from a cosy, warm centrally-heated house into the cold air outside and so into a dramatic change of temperature. Our skin doesn't know where it is. It needs a little help these days.

Here are the basic principles of skin care.

Ideally, everyone, no matter what their skin type, should cleanse, tone and moisturise their face every day.
If you wear no more make-up than lipstick you should still cleanse your face to remove the daily grime, tone the skin to close the pores and moisturise it to keep it young.
If you cleanse your face at night and you are over twenty-five years old it is a good idea to apply a skin food (that is, a night cream).
A moisturiser should be applied in the morning as it is a protector, not a nourisher, and prevents damage to the skin by the elements and provides a good base for any make-up you decide to apply. To ensure you select the best cosmetics for your particular skin, it is necessary for you to diagnose your skin type.

Symptoms of a dry skin are:

1   That it sometimes flakes
2   That it feels taut after washing
3   That it may be very sensitive
4   That it may have a tendency to wrinkling

Symptoms of an oily skin are:

1   A continually shining nose

2   Open pores (giving the appearance of an orange-peel effect on the skin)
3   A tendency towards blackheads and spots

You may consider that your skin is what is commonly known as a 'combination skin'. If your skin is dry on the cheeks, but has an oily patch down the centre of the face, i.e., forehead, nose and chin, then your skin falls into this category.

Cleansing

Ordinary everyday soap can be harmful to the delicate skin on your face. Cosmetic soaps are available but are sometimes very expensive. Preferably find a cleanser to suit your particular skin type. (Combination skin will have to be treated as two separate skin types.)

Apply cleanser with both hands, gently massaging the face in an upward circular movement. This dissolves any make-up or everyday grime and cleanses the pores. Then remove cleanser completely with cotton wool that has been dampened with water and squeezed as dry as possible.

Gently remove all eye make-up with an eye make-up remover lotion, but take care not to drag the skin. Use a non-oily eye make-up cleanser.

Toning

This process not only closes pores which have been opened by the cleanser but it also removes any remaining traces of cleansing cream. Many toning products are available, but there is really no need to spend a lot of money when you can make up your own. Always apply with cotton wool. For a **dry skin** use neat **rose water** (which you can buy from any large chemist).

For an **oily skin** use two parts **rose water** and one part **witch hazel**. This can be made up for you at the chemist or you can buy a bottle of each and mix your own.

For a combination skin use neat **rose water** on dry areas and **rose water and witch hazel** at a 2:1 ratio (as oily skin) on oily centre panel.

Be very careful not to buy a cheap branded product which may be far too astringent for your skin. A toning lotion should not sting the face; if it does, it is too strong.

Night Creams

After thoroughly cleansing and toning your face and neck at night, everyone over the age of twenty-five should apply a small quantity of night cream – one designed for your particular skin type. Ask the advice of a qualified beautician because you want to be sure you buy the correct night cream as they can be expensive.

Apply cream with the tips of the third fingers (these are the most sensitive) and massage gently into the skin. After ten minutes the cream will have penetrated into the face and disappeared. Any excess on the skin will be wasted. It pays to be economical with your night cream.

Moisturisers

A moisturiser should be applied every morning whether you follow it with other cosmetics or not. Even if no other cosmetics are worn a moisturiser is essential. It protects the skin from the elements, and also provides a suitable base on to which a foundation cream may be applied, or alternatively, you may prefer to apply just a little powder.

An **oily skin** needs a cream that is light in texture and non-greasy. It will protect the skin from pollution, thus helping to prevent spots.

A **dry skin** needs a fairly oily moisturiser – one that will protect the skin and remain on the surface to provide a smooth base for your make-up. If the wrong cream is used it will disappear into the skin and you will not be able to apply your foundation cream smoothly.

Combination skins should try using one moisturiser,

applying more to the dry areas. If this is not satisfactory then two separate creams will have to be used.

To sum up

Cleanse and tone every day.

If over twenty-five, feed the skin nightly with a night cream.

Protect your skin every morning with a moisturiser.

Special Creams

There are many creams on the market which are designed for particular problems. These vary from eye creams which can minimise wrinkling and neck creams for the same purpose, to special creams for a dehydrated or tired and generally out-of-condition skin. If you have a particular skin problem it would be money well spent to have a facial by a qualified beauty therapist and to follow her advice. After all we only have one face so we might as well make the most of it!

Face Masks

Depending on your skin type a face mask can help to eliminate spots by thoroughly cleansing the skin. Use according to the instructions described on the particular package. Again, consult your beauty therapist for advice.

Make-up

Each day follow the cleanse, tone and moisturise routine as described under 'Skin Care'.

If you wish to apply make-up, try using your cosmetics in the following order:

Moisturiser Always apply before any make-up as it protects the skin and provides a 'basecoat' or 'undercoat' for your foundation cream, enabling it to be applied smoothly. Apply your moisturiser all over the face and neck with the finger tips using a gentle movement.

Foundation Cream　Foundation cream adds an even-looking colour to your face and can make a tremendous improvement to your appearance. Choose your colour carefully – ask the beauty consultant for advice on shades for your colouring. Apply 'spots' of cream over your face and quickly blend them together with your finger tips, or a damp sponge, extending the movements up to your hairline, ears and neck. Smooth downwards so that the little hairs which are to be found all over your face will lie in the direction in which they grow. Use an old toothbrush to brush out the edges to your hairline and to brush your eyebrows in place. Remember that foundation creams can be mixed to achieve the ideal shade according to the time of year.

Lipstick　Always apply lipstick carefully, preferably with a lip brush (available from chemists or a beauty counter in a larger store). If you wish, you may outline your lips with a lip pencil first. To ensure your lipstick lasts longer, blot the freshly painted lips with a tissue then re-apply.

Blusher　Blusher adds a delightful glow and enhances the shape of your face. Available in powder form or as a cream, apply blusher on the cheekbones and blend in carefully up towards the side of the eyes. If you wish to use face powder, apply cream blusher before the face powder or powdered blusher afterwards. Seek advice from a beautician on suitable shades.

Powder (optional)　Powder helps to set your make-up so that it lasts longer and also helps to provide a matt finish, often desirable for ladies with an oily skin. Apply loose powder with a clean piece of cotton wool. Dab it all over the face pressing rather than rubbing. Brush off excess with cotton wool or a large clean cosmetic brush. Try a translucent shade which is colourless but allows the colour of your foundation to show through.

Eye Base and Shadow   The purpose of eye shadow is to make your eyes appear larger, as well as making them prettier.

Various colours of eye shadow can be combined to create a pretty but subtle effect. For a total eye make-up apply a base of very light shadow (beige or cream) all over the eye area – i.e. from below the eyebrow to above the eyelashes. Then apply a light-coloured eye shadow in the inner corner of the eyelid, and then upwards and outwards with a darker shade. Blend it in carefully. Eye shadows are available in many different forms. Experiment to find which type you prefer: powder, cream or liquid shadow. There are many effective eye foundation creams which prevent creasing and are quite inexpensive.

Eyeliner   This is one cosmetic that is often left out but helps to make your eyes look larger and your lashes thicker.

Apply a thin line next to the upper lashes, from the inner corners to the outer corners. If you wish, you may also apply a very thin line below the lower lashes, but only from the centre outwards (not the full width). There are several excellent eyeliners available which include a very fine brush to ensure easy application. Alternatively, moisten your eye shadow block with a wet eyeliner brush and apply a thin line of moistened shadow close to your lashes. This gives a beautifully natural look, blending in with your eye shadow. Alternatively use one of the new extra-soft eye kohl pencils which can be applied very close to the eyelashes.

Mascara   Apply mascara to upper and lower lashes as desired. A spiral brush ensures easy application separating the lashes while coating them with mascara. This makes them look thicker and longer. Try applying your mascara using zig-zag movements with the brush. This helps separate the lashes and avoids clogging. If you are not used to make-up spend lots of time practising. Only by experimenting will you be able to find the most attractive 'design' for your face.

Make-up should create a beautiful illusion, so try not to overdo it. If you wear glasses, remove them while applying face make-up and lodge them on the end of your nose while you apply your eye make-up.

After completing your make-up you should feel and look much better.

Underwear

Well-fitting underwear can make a tremendous difference to your figure, so it is worth taking a little trouble to find the correct style and size for your particular shape.

A bust need not be flat to warrant a slight padding to give a good shape and uplift and put fullness where it is most needed. Those with heavier bustlines and midriff bulges will find a long-line bra a great help. Very few women wear the correct size bra – they measure themselves around the fullest part of the bustline and hazard a guess as to cup size. Very much a trial and error situation.

The correct way to measure yourself is firstly measure underneath the bust – around the back and ribcage. Add

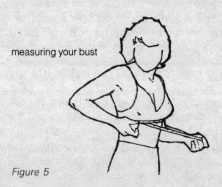

measuring your bust

Figure 5

five inches to that measurement and you will have your correct bra size. For example, if you measure thirty-one inches with the tape measure, add five inches to make it thirty-six inches. You would need a thirty-six-inch bra. Now measure yourself around the fullest part of your bust.

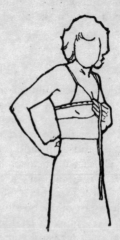

Figure 6

If that measurement is the same as the first measurement (including the five inches) you need a small or A cup; one inch larger indicates a medium or B cup; two inches more indicates a large or C cup; three inches indicates an extra full or D cup.

Always try on a bra before you buy it unless you purchase it from a store which will exchange the garment or refund the money. Pantie girdles can flatten your tummy, but often create huge bulging thighs! You may look better not wearing one at all; in fact I would discourage their use because if they are worn continually thick thighs are almost bound to develop and your waistline will disappear. Similarly, bikini panties if worn too tight, can create bulges on the hips which will remain after they have been removed. Better to buy a size larger brief so they don't cut into the flesh!

Some older ladies find an all-in-one foundation garment a great help. You may be lucky enough to find a make which fits you properly with the bra positioned in the right place. Otherwise you will have to have one made to measure. Alternatively, buy a long-line bra and combine it with a high-line girdle. But again, don't wear one if you can manage without.

To sum up:
Make sure you are wearing the correct size bra for your figure.
Only wear a girdle if you really feel it does something for you – avoid them if possible.
Don't wear panties that are too tight.
If you wish to wear a one-piece foundation garment, make sure that it fits **everywhere**.

Dress sense

Many ladies are unaware that by careful dressing, figure faults can be cleverly camouflaged. Also, the lady who has just become slim after many years of being overweight finds she cannot get used to being slim. She still goes to the size 16 or 18 dresses instead of her proper size of 10 or 12. It is a habit many find difficult to drop.

Here are some simple guide lines.

Always aim to achieve a 'total' look. If your outfit is up-to-the-minute fashionwise then your accessories should be too. Accessories should always match, i.e., black shoes, black handbag, black gloves (though, if you wish, you could wear gloves that are the same colour as your outfit).

Shoes should either match your outfit or be darker. White shoes can be very unflattering unless chosen carefully and worn with a white summer dress or trousers.

Your coat or dress should be the main attraction, with your accessories complementing it. The exception to the rule is, of course, a special hat worn for a wedding, for example. When buying a hat, ask the assistant to demonstrate how it should be worn as few women have the confidence to wear a hat to full advantage.

When shopping for accessories take your outfit with you to compare the colour, suitability, style and so on, and if in any doubt, don't buy!

When choosing something to be worn during the day, judge it in daylight. If it is to be worn in the evening, then make sure that you see yourself in artificial lighting before you decide to buy. Stand back from the mirror and assess the co-ordination of the colours of an outfit at a distance. It is the **general** look which is important.

After a special occasion has taken place, don't put your outfit away never to be worn again until another special occasion. It is too good to waste and as time passes it will become out of date and your figure may change. **Wear it** while it looks at its best and enjoy looking good.

When choosing clothes it helps if you can diagnose your figure type.

There are three categories:

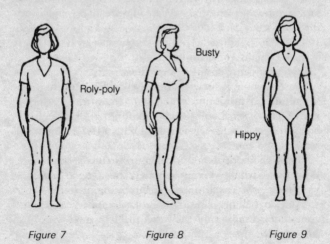

Roly-poly

Busty

Hippy

Figure 7   *Figure 8*   *Figure 9*

Hippy figures look much better in A-line skirts with any patterns or details worn above the waist, not below it. Try to wear darker colours below the waist and light colours or patterns above it.

The reverse applies to busty figures. Often people with heavy busts have delightfully slim hips and legs and look splendid in pleated skirts and in trousers, but they should wear plain dark colours above the waist if they wish to minimise their bust size. Avoid low necklines.

Roly-poly figures should be dressed in plain fabrics and styles should be simple too. No belts, frills or pleats as these only have the effect of making the figure look rounder!

Generally speaking dark colours are more slimming, pastel shades are more flattering to the more mature woman, and if you want to be noticed, wear red. Black and white only accentuate your face so your make-up and hair must be perfect, and avoid these colours if you are feeling under the weather. Wear white- or natural-coloured underwear under white blouses, sweaters and so on. Wear black or natural coloured underwear under black garments, particularly if they are at all see-through.

If you feel the cold try to buy dresses with long sleeves rather than wear a cardigan to keep you warm. A long sleeved dress is much smarter.

Hats are much smarter than headscarves.

Whatever you are wearing should look like an outfit. Don't mix patterns unless they match; always wear a plain blouse with a patterned skirt, and so on. Try not to mix textures either. Wear wool with wool and cotton with cotton.

Plan your wardrobe in advance so that you can make the most of what you buy. It may be a good idea to buy an accessory each time you buy a major item. This way you soon build a wardrobe of accessories enabling you to look really smart all the time.

Nail care

To appear well groomed not only does your hair need to look clean and tidy, your make-up adds something to your beauty, and your clothes help to give the illusion of a perfect figure, but your nails need to look well cared for too.

Nails do not need to be painted to look good. So long as they are the right length and are really clean, they will look fine. If you wish to give yourself a proper manicure your kit should include:

Nail polish remover
A small bowl of warm soapy water and a small towel
An emery board
Cotton wool
Orange stick
Cuticle cream/remover
Hand cream
Base coat (optional)
Nail enamel (optional)
Nail enamel setting oil or an aerosol spray-dry product (optional)

Manicure routine

Assemble everything on a tray
Remove any existing enamel with remover
File nails with an emery board, never a steel file. File in one direction only: towards the centre tip of the nail. Shape the nail into an almond shape.
Wash hands – this removes filings and makes cuticles softer
Dry well
If the cuticles need special attention brush cuticle oil/remover round the cuticles and press back with an orange stick (hoof end) covered with a tiny bit of cotton wool. Remove only dry skin from the cuticle. Never cut your cuticle as it protects the unborn nail which starts at your first knuckle. If the cuticle is cut, germs can creep into this delicate area and cause infection.

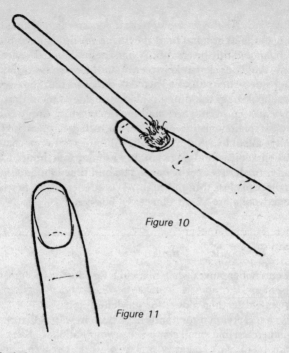

Figure 10

Figure 11

Wash hands again and brush nails. Dry carefully.
Apply plenty of hand cream.
Wipe nails with cotton wool or a tissue to remove all traces
of any grease from the hand cream.
Use nail strengthener at this stage if your nails are brittle,
ask your chemist for advice.
Apply a base coat varnish. This acts as a primer and evens
the surface of the nail. It helps the varnish to stay on better,
and it provides a colourless barrier between your nail and
a dark coloured varnish, thus preventing possible
discolouration by a very strong-coloured enamel.
Apply nail varnish. With hundreds to choose from, find
a shade you really like.
Coat brush with just enough varnish so that it doesn't flood

67

off the end. Re-dip for every nail. If you are right-handed, apply to the right hand first, starting at the little finger and working towards the thumb. If you are left-handed – vice-versa. Apply three strokes to each nail. Centre first, then either side. After painting each nail remove a hairline edge from the nail tip by wiping it along the side of the thumb; this helps to prevent varnish lifting or cracking. Apply two coats of plain varnish or three of frosted or pearlised. Always allow to dry for about five minutes between coats so as to avoid smudging. It takes around four hours for your varnish to set really hard. The best time to manicure your nails is last thing at night. Worst enemies to newly painted nails are sharp objects or hot water.

Tips for hands and nails

Wear rubber gloves when doing the washing or washing up.
Wear old leather gloves for gardening jobs.
Use hand cream after hands have been in water. Carry hand cream in a small container in your handbag. Keep some by the sink and at your place of work. Use as much as your hands will absorb.
Use a thimble when sewing.
Always dry your hands thoroughly – dampness encourages chapping.
If possible give yourself a manicure every week, but leave nails free of varnish for one day each week, so that the air can get to them. Do not remove nail enamel more than once a week as the remover causes drying to the nail surface. If you want to change colour midweek paint a different colour on top of the existing one. Often you can produce some lovely colours by this method.

Deportment and Being Photographed

Many ladies are not sure how to look their best when they are being photographed. It takes practice to look elegant when walking, sitting or standing. Here are some tips.

Standing Stand in front of a mirror and hold your tummy in. Tuck your bottom under and pull your shoulders back. Hold your head up and direct your eyes straight ahead. Now try to keep this position, but relax. See how good you look and how much slimmer you appear!

Walking Imagine that as you walk you are being pulled by two strings that have been threaded through your hip bones. Some model schools teach their models to walk this way. Try to practise this every day and soon it will become natural. Often we stoop, particularly as we get older, and usually this is caused by pushing prams or pushchairs. It is most important to learn to straighten yourself as much

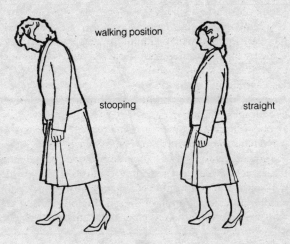

walking position

stooping

straight

Figure 12

as possible. Midriff bulges will disappear and you will look much younger. Practise by walking balancing a book on your head.

Sitting   Sit in front on a full-length mirror. There are three main sitting positions which are considered to be correct. Sit comfortably but upright in the chair.
Position 1 – Feet together but to one side (your big toe joint should fit into the arch of the outer foot) See Figure 13.

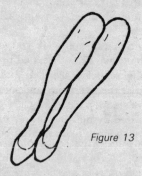

Figure 13

Position 2 – One foot tucked behind the other. Both feet placed to one side. See Figure 14.

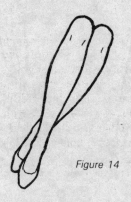

Figure 14

Position 3 – One leg over the other to one side, but knees level (one knee should not be further extended further than the other). The legs should be in line with each other. See Figure 15.

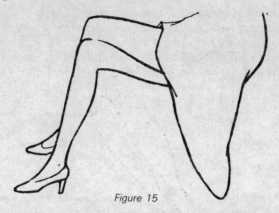

Figure 15

With all these positions, the legs should always be close together and in line with each other. Place your hands together on your lap, the opposite side to your feet.

Photography

General hints worth remembering when being photographed:

1 Never stand straight on at the camera. Stand as we discussed already (standing), but lift one foot half a step backwards and turn the foot out slightly. Swivel the hips a few degrees (in the same direction as the back foot) and this will take inches off your hip width.

2 Slip your handbag over one arm with your arm close to your waist. The other arm should be down by your side. If your bag is a clutch bag, hold it close to your waist, down by your side.

3 White worn next to your face is very flattering on photographs.

71

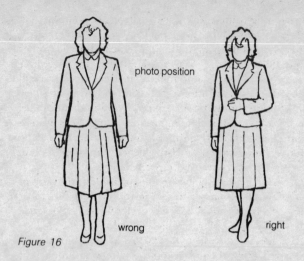

photo position

wrong

right

Figure 16

4 Remember that the person nearest to the camera will look a little larger than the one further away. If you are being photographed with someone who is smaller or slimmer, make sure that they are nearer to the camera!

Personal hygiene

Everyone perspires – some more than others – and most perspiration evaporates quickly and is odourless. It is the stale perspiration that smells unpleasant, either on our bodies or on our clothes, and it can become stale within a few hours by being trapped under our arms and in various other places. If we bathed several times a day, then the chances are that we would not smell. However, it is easier to use a deodorant, which helps to stop odour, although it doesn't prevent wetness. An anti-perspirant attempts to seal in the wetness, thus preventing perspiration in the first place, and therefore the ideal is a deodorant which combines both functions. The extra ingredients will keep you dry as well as odour-free. If you suffer from excessive perspiration, try an extra-strong deodorant. Ask your chemist to advise you.

Often it is not the perspiration that smells, but the clothes that we are wearing. Man-made fibres, in particular polyester and nylon, tend to make you sweat more and will not absorb the perspiration – but as these fabrics are easy to wash, there should be no excuse. Wool and cotton are more absorbent, but still hold the smell. Once perspiration gets into a natural-fibre garment it won't come out, so be careful. Wear a man-made fibre garment for no more than twelve hours under normal circumstances.

We perspire more when anxious or under any kind of stress. Beware of party dresses – we get very warm at parties, so a dress should be worn preferably once, or twice at the very most, before being cleaned.

It is a good idea to spray the palms of your hands with an anti-perspirant if you are about to attend an important function where you may be called to shake hands with many people. Run cold water over your wrists if you wish to cool down quickly.

As well as applying a deodorant and anti-perspirant under you arms you may like to use talc all over your body. This will absorb the moisture and will therefore save your clothes. Apply body lotion after a bath or shower as this will keep your skin soft.

Beware of dark-coloured garments. Just because they don't look dirty doesn't mean they are fresh. You would only wear white once, so wear dark-coloured garments no more than twice.

Experiment with deodorants – there are lots to choose from. Try to find one that really smells good. If you don't like a 'wet' one use a 'dry' one. It is a good idea to carry cologne sachets for a daytime freshen-up. Because we can become immune to one particular brand it is worthwhile changing your deodorant/anti-perspirant every few months.

Menstruation

If you suffer with period pains have a look at what you are eating. Avoid stodgy and sweet things. Do not drink too much alcohol. Vitamin C tablets may help and also a little extra iron in tablet form could be taken.

If the pain continues, consult your doctor. If you feel tired and depressed it could be that you are anaemic.

Be extra careful with hygiene during your periods. Have lots of baths and be extravagant with talc and so on. Avoid using an 'intimate' deodorant – these can do more harm than good and are unnecessary if proper attention is given to personal hygiene.

Take plenty of exercise during your period.

Feet

Wash frequently and for rough skin use a pumice stone, a 'foot scraper' or a branded rough-skin remover cream. Cut toe nails straight across. There are special powders for cooling feet that perspire excessively and foot deodorants are also available.

Body hair

Lip hair can be removed with a depilatory cream, but the instructions on the packet must be followed carefully. Alternatively, you may choose to have your lip waxed by a beautician, but **never** shave your face. Hair under the arms holds perspiration so always remove it, either with a ladies' razor or a depilatory cream, or have it waxed. Hairs on the legs should be removed if they show, and the same depilatory cream could be used. If you must shave your legs don't do so too often as it will create stubble. Waxing is more expensive, but it is a very efficient way of removing hair and discourages growth.

Teeth

Always clean your teeth regularly and carefully. Make a point of seeing the dentist every six months. Try chewing a disclosing tablet (available from any chemist) as this will show up the parts of your teeth which are still unclean. If your breath smells use a mouth freshener. Be careful when you have eaten something strong like garlic or onions, or when you have been a long while without food. Cheese, coffee and milk can also make your breath smell unpleasant.

Hints on grooming

1 Never rush. Don't frown. Keep a mirror in your kitchen to catch you out.
2 The best beauty treatment of all is fresh air, exercise and plenty of sleep.
3 Try to keep up to date and try new styles – they might suit you. Try new hairstyles, but always give a new hairdresser two attempts before judging him or her, as a hairdresser needs to get to know your hair.
4 Always try to wear three colours. The third colour can be jewellery or a scarf, or even matching nail varnish and lipstick.
5 Always be sure to check your back and front in the mirror before going out.

Part 4

Fit for Life

Getting fit, staying fit

One of the most wonderful feelings in the world is getting up in the morning and actually feeling good at the prospect of the day ahead. It is wonderful to be able to feel good whether there is something special to look forward to or whether it just promises to be an ordinary kind of day. If you are feeling fit, relaxed and happy in your mind and content with your body, you can bounce around doing the housework, enjoying the company of your children and smile as your dog chases a butterfly in the garden. You can find that you can cope with your temperamental boss or difficult staff and if you can face the world with a happy smile it's quite amazing how the world really does smile back. It's all a question of energy.

Many people never experience this early morning contented feeling because they have no energy, because they have no *purpose* and they don't feel physically fit. Now I am not talking about training to be an Olympic athlete – that's not what I mean at all. I am talking about going around in our daily lives being able to go up the stairs without puffing and be able to bend down without grunting. Being able to run for a bus or chasing after the dog is a very pleasurable experience if you can do it without feeling you are going to have a seizure when you stop!

Everyone can increase their level of fitness and enjoy a healthy life and almost everyone would be recommended by their doctor to be a little more active if possible. Even those who are restricted to a wheelchair or have only a minimal amount of movement can still find ways of increasing their fitness level, but it does take regular practice. So many potential 'get-fitters' who are completely able-bodied make the mistake of believing that unless their fitness campaign is painful, boring, inconvenient or very expensive, it isn't going to work. They also believe that they must break a world record within the first week of training! Unfortunately, when they don't and they strain a ligament or pull a muscle, they blame the injury for their failure. Achieving fitness is rather like achieving slimness; it takes time and patience. Getting fit doesn't need to involve high-technology equipment nor should it become boring. There is no need for it to be difficult and certainly don't try to be too ambitious. I have met so many people outside of my own classes who have attempted to get fit far too energetically and who have ached so much for the following couple of days or even a week that they have abandoned the whole project on the basis that 'it's not for me'. So it's vital if you are going to get fit that you attempt it in a sensible way.

I was very unfit when I started exercising at my classes back in 1977, but as everyone was recommended to improve their fitness by the Health Education Council when the 'Look After Yourself' campaign was launched, I made the effort to try to be a little more physically active. My experience in physical exercise extended from dancing as a child and practising and training as a Yoga teacher over many of my adult years. I combined the knowledge of both types of exercise and put it to music and this resulted in what I called Slimobility exercises. The fact that these exercises were performed to the latest pop records made it all very enjoyable and soon my class members and I developed a far greater level of fitness and, most

78

important of all, we enjoyed ourselves and were looking forward to the next class.

There are of course a great many different ways of getting fit and in the next few pages you will find exercises to tone up particular parts of your body and to promote stamina and suppleness. Before embarking on any kind of exercise it is wise to check with your doctor first. For instance, anyone with high blood pressure or a heart complaint could benefit from certain exercises but not others so it is essential to check it out first.

Before attempting to exercise for the first time, pause for a moment and realise that you have a network of muscles within the body that resemble large elastic bands. If you found an elastic band in a cupboard that hadn't been used for many years and you stretched it quite hard it would snap very easily. Realise that if you overstretch your body and it has not been worked hard in that way for many years, you too could tear a muscle just as easily. This is where the importance of warming up becomes evident. Returning to the comparison with the rubber band, if you placed the rubber band somewhere warm and gradually manipulated it it would regain its elasticity fairly quickly without causing damage. Similarly, when we embark on exercise – whether it be sport or an exercise session – we must gently warm up all the muscles in our body. The best way to do this is a gentle walking or jogging type movement bringing the arms up and down above your head and generally moving every part of your body in a gentle kind of way, so that you can increase the heart beat and therefore increase the circulation of blood around your body. It is important to realise that the blood pumped around our body keeps us alive.

In a normal sedentary situation it is mostly the main motorways of veins that are used to circulate the necessary oxygen around the body. As soon as we start exercising we need to move more blood around our body more quickly and we do this by opening up the 'A' roads and 'B' roads

79

(smaller veins) so that the blood is circulating everywhere at a far faster pace than normal.

Obviously, if we started too fast doing something that was far too energetic this is where we cause a traffic jam in our veins which can result in angina or heart failure. So, it is vital that every time we are about to exercise we spend at least five minutes warming up our bodies so that our muscles will stretch like a lovely warm rubber band and little damage should be caused.

Exercise for a short time and do not extend the body too far at the beginning of your session. After you have practised your exercises for a while you should not experience any discomfort but instead a feeling of revitalisation. The reason why we sometimes ache after not using our bodies for some considerable time is simply because we work our bodies too hard.

Various muscle tissues are thought to be involved in this aching sensation, but I would need to devote much more space to explain the technicalities of this, so no matter how enthusiastic you may feel towards your fitness campaign, take it gently at the beginning.

Hopefully, after any uncomfortable feeling following an initial workout (usually experienced two days later) you will find that you do not experience similar discomfort again, providing you continue to exercise on a regular basis and at a sensible level. However, it is much more sensible to practise gently and regularly for the first week or so and you will then find yourself working into a really progressive fitness campaign and be able to do more and more without discomfort. You will be delighted at how quickly your body responds as each day goes by and you find that you can perform more exercises with greater ease and with fewer aches the following day.

It must also be realised that our bodies have a natural alarm system in the form of pain. If at any time you feel pain, no matter what kind, you *must* stop exercising immediately. People often think that if they continue 'the pain will go away'. This is dangerous and stupid and we must learn to listen to our bodies. This particularly applies if we are recovering from an illness or operation. But, on the other hand, it is possible to be too cautious in some circumstances when in fact practising light exercise could be helpful as an aid to recovery.

The benefits from exercise are not only that you will look better, but also the condition of your heart will be strengthened and therefore your circulation will improve and thus can help to prevent coronary heart disease. Research has shown that people who take enough exercise can cut their risk of having a heart attack and they may have a better chance of surviving one. Exercise also helps to keep your joints supple as well as your spine and therefore aids in improving posture. Posture is often one of the first signs of ageing years and if you can walk well and upright at eighty you will look many years younger than your age. The Queen Mother is a classic example of this, walking beautifully at such an advanced age. She warms the hearts of the nation because of her youthful looks and endearing personality.

Many people think they are unable to exercise as they reach retirement. I have a lady who attends my slimming and exercise class who is now eighty-three. She has now been attending my classes for over five years. She has shed her three excess stones and joins in all the exercises with the rest of the class and she too is a wonderful incentive for us to try and stay young and energetic.

I mentioned in my introduction the period in my life when I was under a great deal of stress. I found that continuing to take my exercise classes several times a week enabled me to work out my frustration and unhappiness. I honestly think it helped me a great deal to cope under such difficult circumstances.

There are two types of exercise, aerobic and anaerobic. These exercises use different energy systems and are quite different in their activity. Aerobic is where the energy is generated by oxygen breathed in and utilised by our body whereas anaerobic exercise is generated from energy within the body given by food.

Our muscles are made up of two types of fibres. Slow-twitch fibres (red muscle cells) and fast-twitch fibres (white muscle cells). The red-twitch fibres are designed primarily for endurance and stamina work and the white-twitch fibres are designed for speed and strength work.

In order to improve your endurance capability you would therefore do the type of exercises that would involve the red-twitch fibres in work that would improve their endurance capability. This is done by aerobic or stamina-type work which is the sort of exercise now being seen to have the greatest advantages in reducing the risk of heart disease and other associated problems, as well as effectively increasing the metabolic rate – the rate at which we burn up food.

Because of this benefit to our metabolism it is often recommended that slimmers should take some aerobic exercise on a regular basis. To increase your metabolic rate you need to exercise at an activity level which causes your heart to beat significantly faster. You can calculate your personal maximum heart-rate by deducting your age from 220. Calculate 60 per cent and 90 per cent of this number and after a thorough warm-up aim to exercise at an activity level to achieve a heart-rate within these levels. To make sure your heart isn't going over the safety limit (90 per cent) and to ensure that you are working hard enough, you should check your pulse at regular intervals during your aerobic class as well as before and after you begin exercising.

It is important that you take your pulse *immediately* following a maximum activity to find out its effect, as your heart-rate falls rapidly as soon as you stop. At this time count your pulse rate over a six-second period only, and multiply it by ten thus equalling one minute. When checking your pulse rate at rest count over a fifteen second period and multiply by four. For a non-athlete the resting pulse would be usually between sixty and eighty beats per minute. A lower resting pulse rate is generally an indication of fitness, as the heart is pumping the blood around the body more powerfully and efficiently. A top athlete could have a resting pulse rate of between thirty and forty. In order to improve the fitness factor that will be of most benefit to you, that is your aerobic fitness, aerobic exercises are recommended, ideally two or three sessions a week, for twenty to thirty minutes. This will ensure a gradual increase in your fitness level and in your metabolic rate. It may be that you have no wish to go to an exercise class or undertake such a serious check on your fitness level, but the type of aerobic exercise that every able bodied person *can* do, is to go for a really brisk walk three or four times a week for say thirty minutes. This is one of the best forms of exercise we can take being totally safe and good for our all-round health.

Anaerobic activity such as weight lifting, the main purpose of which is strength development, can be of some benefit to your general fitness, but by itself it is a poor way to increase your stamina or endurance levels. So you should look at the activities that give you all-round fitness and the body toning you desire. Try to find an activity that you enjoy so that you will continue doing it long into the future and gain these benefits for the rest of your life. It would be a mistake to undertake a short-term penance that you are quite likely to abandon after achieving your short-term goal. The benefits of regular exercise are so well established now that it should be an integral part of your everyday lifestyle. Just as this book is designed to help you look and feel your best, physical fitness should be a permanent ambition too.

True physical fitness is something more than simply being fit to cope with the stresses and strains of everyday life. It consists of three important ingredients: STAMINA,

Aerobic exercise	Number of calories burned per minute
Badminton – singles	10
– doubles	8
Climbing	12 (approximately)
Cycling	5 to 12 depending on speed
Dancing	3·5 to 8 depending on type
Dance-exercise	5 to 7
Football	9
Gymnastics – moving type	6
Jogging	10 (approximately)
Rowing	11 to 14 depending on speed
Running long distance (e.g. marathons)	11
Tennis	7
Skating	7
Skiing – moderate speed	10 to 16
– uphill, cross country	19
Slimobility exercises	5 to 7
Squash	10
Swimming – breaststroke or backstroke	11 (approximately)
– crawl	14 (approximately)

Anaerobic exercises	Number of calories burned per minute
Discus throwing	3
Golf	5
Gymnastics – strength and balancing type	2 to 4
Weightlifting – heavy weights	4
light weights	2
Yoga	2 (approximately)

SUPPLENESS and STRENGTH – the S-FACTORS as they are commonly called.

First, and perhaps the most important is STAMINA. This is the staying power, endurance, the ability to keep going without gasping for breath. For stamina you need a well-developed circulation in the heart and muscles so that plenty of vital oxygen gets to where it's needed. With stamina you have a slower, more powerful heartbeat. You can cope more easily with prolonged or heavy exertion, and you'll be less likely to suffer from heart disease.

Next is SUPPLENESS or flexibility. You need to develop a maximum range of movements of your neck, spine and joints to avoid spraining ligaments and pulling muscles and tendons. The more mobile you are, the less likely you'll be to suffer from aches and pains brought on by stiffness.

The third S-Factor is STRENGTH, extra muscle-power in reserve for those often unexpected heavier jobs. Moving that sack of potatoes or lifting furniture puts a strain on shoulder, back and thigh muscles. Toned-up tummy muscles also help to take the strain.

The Health Education Council produces many excellent leaflets which explain in more detail the benefits of regular exercise. As a matter of interest I have included the S-Factor scoreboard designed by the Health Education Council which illustrates which activities give you the greatest benefit in this area.

Your choice of exercise must also depend on your general state of health. It is stupid to rush into the sort of vigorous exercise that may aggravate a medical condition. And, of course, it depends on how fit you are already.

When you have selected which type of exercise to take, it is important that the correct clothing is worn, particularly footwear. If you are to attend an aerobic exercise class which includes energetic and continuous movements, the majority of which are on your feet, it is very important

85

	Stamina	Suppleness	Strength
Badminton	**	***	**
Canoeing	***	**	***
Climbing stairs	***	*	**
Cricket	*	**	***
Cycling (hard)	*	***	*
Dancing (ballroom)	*	***	*
Dancing (disco)	***	****	*
Digging (garden)	***	**	****
Football	***	***	***
Golf	*	**	*
Gymnastics	**	****	***
Hill walking	***	*	**
Housework (moderate)	*	**	*
Jogging	****	**	**
Judo	**	****	**
Mowing lawn by hand	**	*	***
Rowing	****	**	****
Sailing	***	***	**
Squash	***	***	**
Swimming (hard)	****	****	****
Tennis	**	***	**
Walking (briskly)	**	*	*
Weightlifting	*	*	****
Yoga	*	****	*

*   No real effect
**   Beneficial effect
***   Very good effect
****   Excellent effect

By permission of the Health Education Council

to wear proper aerobic exercise shoes which include a cushioning sole. This helps to cushion the jarring of your legs, particularly if you are exercising on a very hard floor. Don't be deceived by a nice carpet on the top. Underneath it could be concrete and this could be quite harmful to your legs. If you exercise perhaps only once or twice a week and are on a wooden 'sprung' floor, then it may not be necessary for you to use special shoes. It is always a good idea to wear leg-warmers too. These help to prevent muscle strain as they keep your calves and ankles warm. If you do feel energetic enough to go jogging outside, always remember to jog on grass whenever possible as it is much too tough on the legs to jog on the pavements or roads. For jogging it is also absolutely essential that you wear suitable shoes and not just an old pair of plimsolls that you have in the cupboard. Proper jogging shoes will save you an awful lot of pain later on. If you want to start jogging then it's a good idea to do so by combining alternate jogging and walking for a maximum of fifteen minutes on the first outing and gradually increasing the jogging and decreasing the amount you walk each day following. When you can jog continuously for fifteen minutes you will be ready to increase your distance.

When undertaking any kind of bending or stretching exercise it is advisable to wear a leotard or catsuit or a loose-fitting jogging outfit or tracksuit. The waistband should never be too tight as this will cause discomfort during your exercises. Loose and comfortably fitting shorts and a sweatshirt or teeshirt are also idea for most sporting activities.

One of the most beneficial forms of exercise for anyone with any kind of disability or who suffers from painful arthritic or rheumatic complaints, or perhaps is just recovering from surgery, is to do so in water. You don't have to be a good swimmer to enjoy the benefits of exercising in the weightlessness of a swimming pool. Exercising under water adds a completely new dimension

Aerobic exercises

These exercises are for a general all over warm-up.
Practise to bouncy music and repeat each exercise
at least ten times.

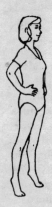

Toe raises

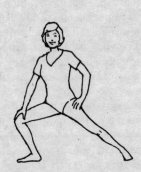

Side lunges
each side

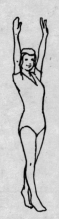

Walking tall

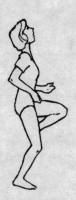

Jogging

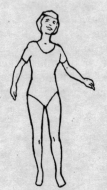

Jogging
side to side

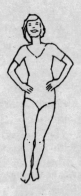

Side jumps
from side
to side

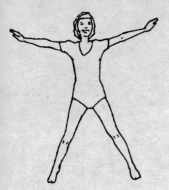

Leg split jumps out

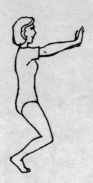

Bounce
the knees

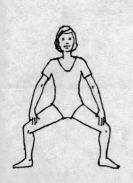

With knees apart
bounce centrally

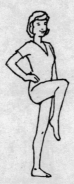

Raise knees
across with
alternate legs

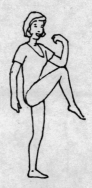

Then increase
movement to
touch elbow
to knee

Figure 17

Spot-reducing exercises

For the arms, bust and shoulders
Practise to any music with a 4/4 tempo. Repeat
each movement at least 10 times.

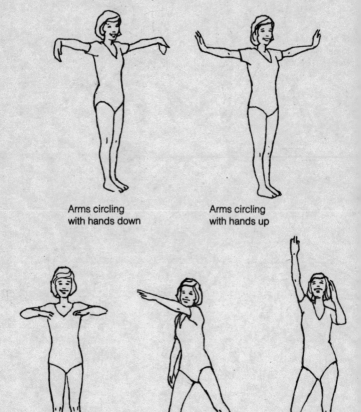

Arms circling
with hands down

Arms circling
with hands up

Elbow thrusts
forward and back
Figure 18

Arms swinging and circling to each side
Make as wide a circle as possible

Reach up
really high
10 times

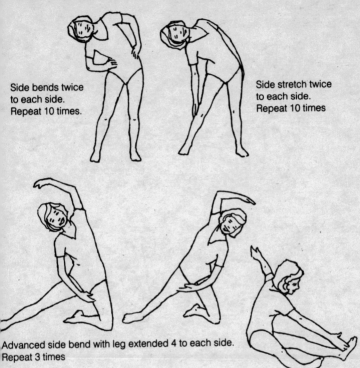

Side bends twice
to each side.
Repeat 10 times.

Side stretch twice
to each side.
Repeat 10 times

Advanced side bend with leg extended 4 to each side.
Repeat 3 times

With arms far apart
slap alternate feet

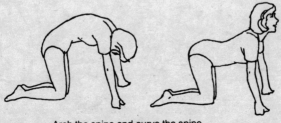

Arch the spine and curve the spine

Figure 19

For thighs, hips and buttocks
Repeat each exercise 10 times and practise to
fast-tempo music.

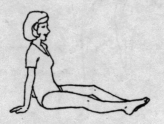

Leg bounces, fast

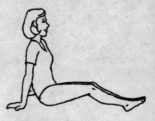

Bounce both legs
together

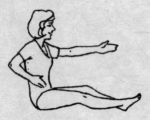

Bottom walking
10 steps forward,
10 back

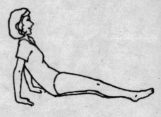

Bottom bounces

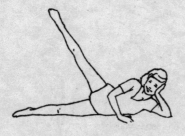

Leg raises

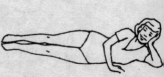

and together

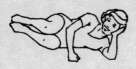

Knee bends and stretch

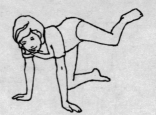

Raise bent leg sideways

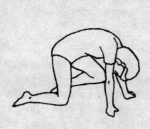

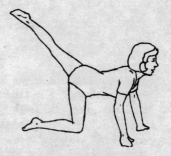

Relax your head down and bring your knee towards your chin,
then extend leg and raise head

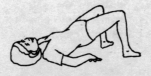

Using your arms and hands to
support you, raise your hips and
then squeeze knee muscles without
altering the position of your legs

Figure 20

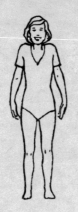

Shoulder circling.
10 backward
and 10 forward

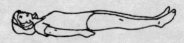

Slowly lie down and relax completely for
5 to 10 minutes

Figure 21

to normal exercise as the limbs are worked against the
weight of the water and therefore the body works harder.
It is also quite hard work keeping your balance, but on
the other hand you can enjoy the beautiful feeling of
weightlessness. For this reason many disabled people find
water exercise very useful. In the following pages I give
some examples of some water exercises.

Waist exercises

1 Hands on hips. Twist 20 times ensuring that your
  elbows are well below the water.
2 Hands on hips, swivel your hips in an anticlockwise and
  clockwise direction 10 each way.

Leg and hip exercises

1 Hold on to the edge of the pool with your right hand.
  Swing your left leg, keeping it straight, forward and
  backward like a ballet dancer. After 10 repetitions with

94

your left leg, turn round and swing your right leg 10 times.

2 Standing in the pool to chest level, raise alternate legs in front of you and touch your foot with your hand. Alternate legs and arms and touch 20 times in total.

3 Holding on to the pool rail facing inwards towards the centre of the pool, draw as big a circle as possible with alternate legs. Practise circling 20 times – 10 each leg.

4 Jog on the spot with water at chest level. 20 steps in total.

5 Jump and allow legs to separate as wide as possible as you land. Arms should go outward too to perform a water jumping-jack. Jump with feet together again and hands down by your side. Perform 10 times.

6 Instead of separating your legs sideways as in 5 perform leg and arm split jumps to the front and back, but do not stop as they come together in the middle. Just jump all the time to allow your legs to go from front to back without a break, and swing your arms forward and backward too. Perform 10 times.

7 Stand as far as possible away from the pool bar, but near enough to hold on to it with your hands. Stretch one straight leg up toward your hands leaving the other stretched well out behind you. Change legs after holding the position for 4 seconds. Repeat 10 times with each leg.

Arm exercises

1 Stand in the pool so that your shoulders are just submerged in the water. Bend your arms below water level and thrust your elbows back 20 times.

2 Make a paddle with both hands and try to push the water aside as you work them from left to right, 10 times each way. Arms must be straight throughout the exercise.

3 Standing in water at a level just below the shoulders, swing straight arms together in circles. Firstly, make circles backwards 10 times and then reverse the direction and perform 10 times forwards.

95

Maintaining our slimming success is often considered much more difficult than actually losing weight in the first place. Most dieters find it fairly straightforward to follow a diet restricting their intake of calories and achieving a reduction. But when a restriction is lifted and we are given a certain amount of freedom to choose which particular foods we fancy, many slimmers find it very difficult to exercise moderation in either their selection or quantity of food they are now allowed to consume. It's almost as though under the restriction of the diet the rules are very straightforward and we can stick to them, but as soon as they are lifted our freedom goes to our head!

Because my Hip and Thigh Diet broke through a lot of the barriers of no calorie counting and very little weighing of food, slimmers found it easier to maintain their new weight, because those rules didn't seem to be quite as strict. However, no matter which diet you might have followed, the laws of weight maintenance remain the same. The secret is to return to non-diet normal eating in stages. If you return to eating fish and chips, steak and chips and egg and bacon after following any kind of diet you will obviously regain your weight in no time. On the other hand, if you introduce any of these things occasionally you will find that you are able to enjoy them with a clear conscience without the feeling of being paranoid about regaining all your lost weight.

The key to maintaining a lower weight is simply eating sensible foods in moderate quantities. If you have lost weight on food which has been satisfying then it is easier to adjust, but if you have lost weight on starvation rations the adjustment requires more patience. However, there is no doubt it can be achieved just the same.

Generally speaking, the ideal way to adjust after losing weight is to just slightly increase the quantities of the foods you enjoy most and to keep an eye on the scales and the tape measure to judge whether they are in fact causing you to gain weight or not. You will soon get a feel for which foods you can eat freely without weight gain, and which foods you have to restrict or eat only occasionally.

If you have been following a diet and have no idea what your metabolic rate is now, it could be worthwhile testing it for a week by recording every mouthful of food that you eat or drink and to add up the calories at the end of the week to see what your total consumption has been. Remember to weigh yourself at the commencement of your seven-day record and of course again a week later. If, after following a fairly normal eating pattern for seven days you find that your weight has remained the same, then it is clear that the number of calories you have consumed is ideal for you at the moment. If, on the other hand, you lost weight then you can increase your calories or if you gained weight then obviously you ate more calories than your body burned up, and the necessary adjustment must therefore be made. I give on the next page an ideal way to list your calories intake for a week together with columns for you to record the calorie values of each item.

Of course, the other way you can help to maintain your weight is to increase the amount of exercise that you do. As I have said earlier in this book, if we can use up more calories in exercise then we are able to consume more in food if we so wish. The choice really is yours. Personally, I have a very large appetite and I find it easier to do extra exercises and still be able to eat the food that I love rather than cut down on the food and do less physical activity. It is obviously all a question of personal choice and arriving at a balance to suit your individual needs.

Over a period of time you will gain confidence in your control of your weight and of your food consumption. If you are going out for a special meal and you know that you are going to probably have two days' calories in one sitting, it is always a good idea to cut down the day before you go and indeed during the early part of the day of the

	Monday	Cals	Tuesday	Cals	Wednesday	Cals	Thursday	Cals	Friday	Cals	Saturday	Cals	Sunday	Cals
Breakfast														
Mid-morning														
Lunch														
Mid-afternoon														
Evening Meal														
Supper														
TOTALS														

special meal. Also, skip breakfast the following day and perhaps have a light lunch. This way you will be able to correct any 'damage' that may have been caused by the exceptional treat of the night before. When keeping an eye on your weight during your maintenance trial period do remember that just prior to menstruation many women gain weight, so don't let this cause a false reading on the scales. Perhaps try out your maintenance programme just after your period.

It is important to realise how very hard you have been working to lose your unwanted pounds and how good it is to feel so much slimmer. The extraordinary thing is that many slimmers, having achieved a much slimmer figure, often become very critical of their new shape. 'But I've still got a big tummy' or 'I've still got huge thighs' are typical moans from people who have lost lots of weight but still feel there is some to lose in specific areas. It is a shame that not every slimmer takes a photograph of themselves before they commence the diet, because if they did and they were able to look at it frequently they would soon realise what a tremendous achievement they have made. We should not be so self-critical and we must realise that in our eyes we never will be perfect. Whilst this is perhaps little consolation when we are striving to improve our outward appearance, we must take comfort from the fact that even those who we would look upon as having perfect figures would consider themselves far from perfect if you were to ask them. So don't belittle your achievement and appreciate the success that you *have* achieved and enjoy it!

Part 5

Successful Living

Successful living can only be achieved if you are happy. So what is happiness? I believe it is waking up in the morning feeling glad that it is another day. Having a warm feeling in your heart – a feeling that you are at peace with yourself and with your life. If you have not yet experienced these beautiful feelings I want to show you how you can. I believe that life should be an exciting adventure and that everything that happens in it – good and bad – is for our benefit. Let me explain.

We must realise that everyone of us is an individual and we must accept that we have our own character and personality. Some people are more ambitious than others and they will experience greater excitement and anxiety than those more content to just drift along. The entrepreneur won't be happy unless his next project is about to get off the ground. He will lie in bed at night, his mind alive with ideas. The variety in his life prevents boredom and his determination to succeed will enable him to win more than he loses. If every idea succeeded he would become more and more ambitious, taking greater risks because it is the chance that he might fail that makes his life exciting. On the other hand, some people prefer to be more cautious. They choose a steady job with a regular income and are quite happy to settle for less, knowing that at least they are secure. There is absolutely nothing wrong with either situation, as long as both parties are happy.

If getting up in the morning is a real pain, there is definitely something wrong. Many people are unhappy because of something in their everyday life and I believe that life is rather like a garden. Within the garden we have flowers and the inevitable weeds. In some gardens of life there are more weeds than flowers and I believe that we should always remove these, one by one, and plant in their place some beautiful flowers. What I am trying to say is that if in your life you've got a problem at work – perhaps a difficult colleague – or a problem with a difficult neighbour, I suggest that you face the problem head-on and try to sort it out. I never cease to be amazed how easily huge problems can be resolved so simply if they are faced head-on as early as possible. Problems play on our minds and often become exaggerated and out of all proportion, because they are left to fester.

Let's take an example of a situation arising between two families living next door to each other. One day the young daughter of family 'A' – (Louise aged 7) – has been asked to take some flowers to school for a nature lesson. Louise doesn't have any flowers in her garden and so pops in next door and helps herself to some pretty flowers out of the garden belonging to family 'B'. Louise walks into her house and shows her mother her newly acquired blooms and her mother says, 'Where did you get those from?' Louise says, 'I borrowed them from next door'.

Mother is devastated by her daughter's actions and immediately explains to the daughter that she shouldn't have gone next door and that when she goes to school she mustn't tell anyone where she picked the flowers from. Mrs 'A' is now worried to death that Mrs 'B' will accuse her daughter of being a thief. She's immediately on the defensive every time Mrs 'B' comes anywhere near. In fact, she hides behind the curtain if she thinks Mrs 'B' is going past her front door and avoids Mrs 'B' at all costs whenever possible. Before we know where we are Mrs 'B' thinks 'Well I don't know what I've done to upset Mrs 'A', but

I've obviously done something, so I had better keep out of the way', and a family rift is now well and truly developing. Wouldn't it have been better if Mrs 'A' had gone round immediately to Mrs 'B' and said, 'I am terribly sorry but Louise has picked some of your flowers for a Biology lesson. I've told her she shouldn't have done and I really cannot apologise enough.' Mrs 'B' would have to be inhuman not to accept such an apology, particularly if it was done instantly. No further problems would have developed and everything would have been forgotten and life could have continued.

This is just an example of the type of situation which happens in our lives many times a week. If we face it head-on, immediately, often the problem can be sorted out very painlessly without any detriment to anyone. In fact, often relationships can even be improved by such honesty.

I find when I am faced with a difficult situation that I always ask the Lord for direction. Often, within minutes a situation has unfolded where I can easily approach the problem. I also take to the Lord any questions where I am not sure which way to turn. I talk to Him as though He was my best friend (which He is of course) and He is able to show me which is the right way to go.

We need our own ideas and dreams and there is nothing but good to come out of having a goal. Having a goal is being able to achieve something and give you the personal feeling of satisfaction. The goal can be anything from climbing a mountain to raising a lot of money for your favourite charity. It can be a business goal or a personal goal, but whatever it is it is giving you an aim and that must be good. But we need to exercise total determination and the energy with which to realise that goal.

Unfortunately, most people never achieve their true potential because they just don't think. They conform with society and wander aimlessly through their lives getting absolutely nowhere. I was once told a story that illustrated exactly this problem. If we take two identical ships situated in a harbour, one has a captain and crew and the other does not. The captain knows his destination precisely and has his route carefully planned. He's been planning it for some time and he is virtually certain to reach his destination. The other ship does not have a captain or a crew and has no particular place to go. It drifts helplessly around, being blown by the wind and the tides and bumping into things and getting absolutely nowhere. A lot of people are like that. They go through the education system, find a job – often any job they can get just so that it gives them some money – they then perhaps meet someone and marry them and maybe have children and then just drift through the rest of their lives. This is incredibly sad, because life becomes one big struggle to make ends meet and they often are burdened with envy at those around them who seem to have their lives better organised. Often these people feel that life has passed them by and they even feel cheated. We have to work hard at our lives to improve them, to value the gifts we have been given and use them wisely and well. Only we can help ourselves to do this, and it is often easier to feel sorry for ourselves than to try to improve our life and that of others. We must try to be thoughtful to others and help to make everyone's life as pleasant as possible.

When I first became a Christian I read a little book for new Christians which explained that making a prayer list was a good idea. I bought a little notebook, and I listed the various things that I prayed for. This would include everything from my dog's paw getting better and that the lady in our local shop would recover from cancer to my over-eating becoming controlled, that my marriage would continue to be happy, my daughter would be protected and be safe, and that we could have a new car next year! As the months go by, I add new requests to the list and tick those that have been granted. It is quite staggering to see how 99 per cent of the things that have been asked for have been given. I feel that if I ask God for help then He will give it and that He does want me to be happy.

'SEEK and you shall find' is so true in our life. Often we expect things to just fall into our laps, rather than go out looking for them. There are times in our lives when we must go looking, whether it be for a job or an item for the home or for help. Often the thing that we are searching for is right under our noses. We somehow need to have the courage to go out and look, and to keep on looking for what we want, and not to give up.

It is always interesting to hear of the television presenter or the pop star who from a very early age made themselves a total nuisance in the particular career that they wanted to venture into. They didn't *start* as a television presenter or a pop star. Only by asking, seeking and continually trying, were they at last listened to and given the opportunity that allowed them to achieve their aim. I also think that the Lord sometimes places the occasional obstacle along the way so that we can actually take stock and decide whether or not we really *do* want what we are asking. I have seen this situation happen so often in my life. Just before I make a final decision, perhaps buying a house or whatever, I would look back and take stock of the pros and cons of the situation. Weighing up the advantages and disadvantages, I might say, 'Yes, all right, the situation has its disadvantages but I still want to do it.' At that point of making the decision I feel a great sense of determination and the Lord seems to step in and offers real help.

In this book I have been talking about having a personal goal and achieving happiness, both of which I believe cannot be achieved without God's help. Success is to do with personal happiness and fulfilment. It is being happy doing your particular type of work and feeling fulfilled. People often say to me, 'Well, that's all very well if you know what you want to do, but I don't know what I want to do to be happy.' I sympathise with this situation and have witnessed many people who basically haven't got any idea what their main goal is. A lot of people make excuses as to why they can't do this or that, and why they are not cut out to be successful. We should try to eliminate excuses altogether and we should also eliminate the words 'I can't' from our vocabulary. We must realise that it is our desire, not our ability, that determines our success. If we want to do something badly enough we are almost certain to achieve it, it is God's wish too.

I think it is vital to develop a positive mental attitude and this can be done by trying to see the best in every situation. Instead of criticising or being negative, try and look at the good side of people and compliment them when they have done something well or have made an effort. I find paying someone a compliment makes them positively shine and this develops such a delightfully happy atmosphere. No-one is above being complimented whether it be on their appearance or on a job well done. It has such a positive effect that it only brings the best out of that person as they continue in whatever direction they are working towards.

I believe we should build up a defence mechanism to protect us from negative people. Jesus never allowed those who criticised him to upset Him. He never defended himself or tried to explain why they were wrong. He just told positive parables to explain His point of view. He just turned the other cheek, never rising to their bait.

I have learned to listen to the Lord's advice over everything. I don't always like it but I find it is easier in the end because the Lord ALWAYS wins! Sometimes when I ask for guidance on something He says, 'Wait' and I have to be patient. Sometimes He says, 'No' but usually when He does say 'No' it is because He is saying, 'There is something better that I have in mind for you.' How many times have you spotted the house or car or job of your dreams only to lose it to someone else? We feel desperately disappointed at the time. It seems at the time that it was *exactly* what we were looking for. But we find a better house, car or job and we say, 'It all worked out for the best in the end'.

One of the greatest lessons I learned from the Lord was that of trusting Him with my life. Let me explain. If we imagine a bird migrating, we realise that he flaps his wings to get started on his long journey, to change position, or to speed things up a bit. However, most of the time he drifts along on the thermals, effortlessly gliding for miles and miles. I believe life should be like that. We shouldn't flap our wings all the time but let the Lord show us what to do in every situation. There are times when I feel overwhelmed by the mountain of jobs waiting to be done – books to be completed, TV scripts to write, deadlines to meet. . . . Yet, if I place the whole lot in the hands of the Lord and say, 'Please show me how to cope' He *always* does. It is quite incredible how much work does get done and on time!

Human nature is very strange. We tend to mess around trying out our ideas to solve our problems rather than ask for help to sort them out. We waste so much time and energy. I think it is a good idea to keep a diary, to record times when we've had encourgement. On a bad day, it is good to be able to look back at all that we have achieved. It makes us feel better and lifts us out of the doldrums. So let us finish on a note of glorious optimism. Life's garden should be full of beautiful flowers – full of things that give us pleasure and love. If you don't have a partner, or a family living with you, perhaps think about getting a cat or a dog. They help to give us a purpose to the day and it's also very therapeutic to physically stroke a pet. We all need to love and be loved. Success is our ability to achieve our goals in life. It has nothing at all to do with being wealthy or being academically clever; anyone can have this fulfilment and I hope this book will help you to achieve it. May God bless you richly.

Extra help is available

Rosemary Conley's
HIP AND THIGH EXERCISE CASSETTE AND POSTER

You'll love what it does for you!

Now you can feel fitter, healthier and even more fabulous with the fun-fitness exercise programme specifically designed to tone your hips and thighs.

This energetic but easy to follow exercise workout, to your favourite pop music, has been written and presented by Rosemary Conley. It is specially designed to tone you up as you lose your weight and inches on the Hip and Thigh Diet and will help you to keep your new trim figure toned for ever. The cassette comes with fully illustrated instructions at £5.99 inclusive of postage and packing. (UK and Northern Ireland only.)

Rosemary Conley's
HIP AND THIGH VIDEO

Rosemary Conley's Hip and Thigh Video offers personal advice to followers of her Hip and Thigh Diet. You can learn how to cut out the fat in the kitchen, how to defeat temptation and how to cope with the difficult times!

Also you can work out with Rosemary in the comfort of your own home with the Hip and Thigh Exercise Programme, specifically designed to tone your hips and thighs as you lose your weight and inches. This is the fun way to get fit and to keep your new trim figure toned for ever.

The video is written and presented by Rosemary Conley and is available on VHS price £9.99 including postage and packing. (Available in the U.K. and Northern Ireland only.)

Rosemary Conley's
HIP AND THIGH POSTAL SLIMMING CLUB

Rosemary Conley received many letters from readers asking for details of a club where they could find personal help and support whilst following her Hip and Thigh Diet. The Postal Slimming Club offers that personal advice and encouragement from experienced Slimming Consultants.

The initial eight-week course costs £13.99 and this can be extended to suit your individual needs as required. For further details and an enrolment form, without obligation, please write to Rosemary Conley's Postal Slimming Course, Dept LG, PO Box 4, Mountsorrel, Loughborough, Leicestershire LE12 7LB enclosing a stamped, self-addressed envelope. (Available in the UK and Northern Ireland only.)

ORDER FORM

Please supply:

	Quantity	Total £
Audio cassette(s) and Posters @ £5.99 each	_____	_____
Video cassette(s) @ £9.99 each	_____	_____
	TOTAL	_____

*I enclose a cheque/P.O. for £*_____

Please send me details of your Postal Slimming Course

☐ *Please tick*

Please complete in block capitals:

NAME: _____

(MR, MRS, MS, MISS)

ADDRESS: _____

_____

POSTCODE: _____

Prices include postage and packing. All cheques should be made payable to Rosemary Conley Mail Order A/C. *Please write your name and address on the reverse of the cheque* and allow 21 days for delivery. Please send the above coupon with your remittance, to:

Rosemary Conley Enterprises, Dept LG,
PO Box 4, Mountsorrel, Loughborough,
Leicestershire LE12 7LB